OUTCOMES OF EFFECTIVE MANAGEMENT PRACTICE

SONA

SERIES ON NURSING ADMINISTRATION

An annual publication planned and administered by the University of Iowa, **SONA** addresses current and emerging issues in nursing administration. In each volume, distinguished nurse administrators and educators address the state of knowledge, future directions, and controversial questions on aspects of a particular issue and propose options for resolution. The series provides a quality resource for practicing administrators, faculty teaching nursing administration, and students in administration programs.

OUTCOMES OF EFFECTIVE MANAGEMENT PRACTICE

Kathleen Kelly
Editor

Meridean Maas
Chair of the Board

SONA 8

Series on Nursing Administration

SAGE Publications
International Educational and Professional Publisher
Thousand Oaks   London   New Delhi

For information address:

SAGE Publications, Inc.
2455 Teller Road
Thousand Oaks, California 91320
E-mail: order@sagepub.com

SAGE Publications Ltd.
6 Bonhill Street
London EC2A 4PU
United Kingdom

SAGE Publications India Pvt. Ltd.
M-32 Market
Greater Kailash I
New Delhi 110 048 India

Printed in the United States of America

Library of Congress Cataloging-in-Publication Data

Main entry under title:
Outcomes of effective management practice / editor, Kathleen Kelly;
    chair of the board, Meridean Maas.
        p. cm.—(Series on nursing administration; v. 8)
    Includes bibliographical references and index.
    ISBN 0-8039-7175-3 (cloth: acid-free paper)
        1. Nursing services—Administration—Evaluation. 2. Outcome
assessment (Medical care) 3. Nursing services—Evaluation.
    I. Kelly, Kathleen. II. Maas, Meridean. III. Series.
RT89.098   1996
362.1'73'0685—dc20   95-32517

This book is printed on acid-free paper.

99 10 9 8 7 6 5 4 3 2

Production Editor: Diane S. Foster

Contents

Series Preface

Today's nurse executive needs to stay current in many rapidly changing areas of health care. To meet this demand, the **Series on Nursing Administration** is designed to give nursing administrators new information on current and emerging issues. Developed and managed at the University of Iowa College of Nursing and published by Sage, it is a quality resource for nurse executives, faculty who teach nursing administration, and students in nursing administration programs. Each year a new volume addresses the most recent issues in this discipline. Thus a subscription to the series will keep readers on the forefront of knowledge and practice.

Every nurse executive interacts with corporate management; colleagues in other settings, professional groups, the community, and clients; and nurse colleagues, members of other disciplines, and ancillary personnel. To stay current with developments in each of these areas, the nurse executive reads journals and newsletters, attends continuing education programs, and partici-pates in short-term executive management courses. The most effective method, however, is the sharing of concerns, experiences, and insights with peers. The Sage **Series on Nursing Administration** formalizes the process of sharing among experts with similar concerns. In every chapter of each volume of the series, expert authors share their experiences and ideas on particular emerging issues. Busy nurse executives can conveniently and cost-effectively keep their knowledge current on a variety of topics by reading this series.

Nursing administration faculty can use the series to keep their teaching and practice alive, current, and timely. Most nursing administration programs have one or more courses that address issues in nursing management. Because these issues undergo rapid change, faculty need a flexible approach to teaching this content. This series offers the instructor maximum flexibility in selecting issues for discussion to fit the needs of a particular class. An instructor teaching a nursing management issues course can use the series as a course text. Students introduced to it will find it a resource with ongoing value. Faculty teaching undergraduate-level administration courses also may use the series to supplement an introductory text on management and leadership.

The series is unique in that it is the first annual series devoted to issues in nursing administration. To ensure that it covers current issues and provides up-to-date information, the series employs a unique publication process involving four groups: a series editor, an editorial board, the authors, and the publisher.

Editor of Volumes 1 through 4 of the series is Marion R. Johnson, RN, PhD, an assistant professor at the University of Iowa. She has a rich practice base in nursing administration and currently teaches nursing administration at the master's level. Her background, interests, and writing skills made her eminently qualified for the job of series editor.

Kathleen Kelly, PhD, RN, is the editor for Volumes 5 through 8 of the series. She has years of experience as a community health nursing administrator and teaches nursing administration at the master's level. She also administers the Continuing Education Program at the College of Nursing. Her background and current work provide a broad perspective on issues that are of critical importance to nurse executives and managers.

Sue Moorhead, PhD, RN, is the editor starting with Volume 9. She has years of experience in administration as an army nurse and currently is an assistant professor at the University of Iowa. The military provided her with a diverse clinical background and a broad perspective of administrative issues in nursing. She currently teaches undergraduate students at the College of Nursing.

The editorial board consists of faculty teaching in the nursing administration program at Iowa and selected nurse administrators associated with the program. The board meets three or four times a year with the series editor, helps identify the emerging issues and prospective authors, and assists the editor with manuscript review. Iowa's growing program in nursing administration, including study at the doctoral level, makes the University of Iowa an ideal setting to support this publication. A National Advisory Board consisting of nursing administrators, both academic and practicing, advises the editorial board on pertinent topics and authors where needed.

The authors are distinguished nurse administrators, educators, and researchers chosen for their expertise in particular areas. Although authors have the freedom to pursue an issue as they choose, each is encouraged to address the state of knowledge, future directions, and controversial questions surrounding the issue and to propose one or more options for resolution. Beginning with Volume 7, authors were chosen by a review process following a call for abstracts. The call for abstracts is mailed and advertised in various journals and newsletters during the months of February through September each year.

The publisher of the series, beginning with Volume 7, is Sage Publications, Inc. Mosby Year Book, Inc., published Volumes 3 through 6, and Volumes 1 and 2 were published by Addison-Wesley.

All of us involved in this series believe that it will benefit not only those who teach and practice nursing administration but the entire nursing profession and, most important, the patients we serve. We welcome your comments and suggestions.

Diane Gardner Huber, PhD, RN, FAAN
Chairperson, Editorial Board, Volumes 9-10

Meridean L. Maas, PhD, RN, FAAN
Chairperson, Editorial Board, Volumes 5-8

Joanne Comi McCloskey, PhD, RN, FAAN
Chairperson, Editorial Board, Volumes 1-4

Introduction

The eighth volume of the **Series on Nursing Administration** (SONA) captures the state of scientific investigation and practice related to outcomes of effective management practice. The focus on outcomes is a local progression from previous volumes that have focused on structure and process aspects of management of health care and the systems in which they are delivered. It provides readers with cutting-edge thinking and organizational efforts to define and classify outcomes, test approaches to outcomes management, apply outcomes management concepts in various practice settings, and integrate various outcomes-related research into health care practice and management. The work shared by Volume 8 contributors is offered to provoke critical thinking about outcomes of health care and the contribution that management intervention can make to achieving desired outcomes. This is the ultimate measure of effective management interventions.

Volume 8 has particular relevance for nurses and other providers with responsibilities for clinical care management and for those in systems management roles. It is organized in three parts, and as the part introductions demonstrate, the content of many chapters has both clinical care management and systems management applications. Not since Volume 5, *Managing Nursing Care,* has SONA integrated clinical practice and management issues so consistently. The title was chosen to reflect the interrelationship of outcomes and management practice. The content of chapters reflects the scope of outcomes that are being addressed by leaders in outcomes research and practice.

Part 1 of Volume 8 provides a framework for viewing the concepts and issues that link health care outcomes and management practice. In addition to exploring systems issues of uniform language development and systematic evaluation of interventions, authors provide an overview of outcomes issues related to ongoing health care reform and trends toward ambulatory care. This section includes nursing perspectives on one of the most highly publicized outcomes research programs—The Medical Outcomes Studies (MOS)—focusing on one of the program's outcomes measurement instruments, the SF-36.

With Part 1 as a background, Part 2 addresses process or methodological issues associated with outcomes measurement and management. Such timely topics as variance tracking and analyses, implementing AHCPR clinical guidelines, and implications for case management and managed care are featured here. The topic of creative staff scheduling and the impact on nursing practice outcomes rounds out this section.

Part 3 offers five chapters that focus on evaluation of outcomes management in a variety of settings. Authors share their knowledge and experience gained through program development, implementation, and evaluation. Reports range from implementing advanced nursing practice in the neonatal intensive care setting to evaluating outcomes of long-term care in institutional and noninstitutional settings. Outcomes measures reported by authors include cost, satisfaction and clinical status of clients, and provider satisfaction. Specific management practices evaluated in these chapters include implementation of advance nursing practice in neonatology; evaluation of nurse-managed care employing clinical pathways in long-term care settings; multidisciplinary case management employing clinical pathways in a rehabilitation unit; strategies of evaluating cost outcomes in an inpatient, acute care setting; and implementation of a broad-based work redesign program in the acute care setting.

Each section of this volume integrates applied research, clinical and management practice, and futuristic thinking about health care outcomes. This volume demonstrates how effective management practice will contribute to achieving outcomes that serve the priorities of consumers of care, payers, health care providers, and the organizations that provide structure for the delivery of health care services. Health care providers and managers, educators, and researchers will value this publication for its linking of theory and practice in one of the major health care concerns of the decade—managing outcomes of effective management practice.

Kathleen C. Kelly, PhD, RN

A Framework for Linking Management Interventions and Health Care Outcomes

Part 1 provides a framework for viewing the issues and concepts linking management interventions with health care outcomes. The authors represent experienced clinicians, managers, and researchers. The combined work of these authors sets the stage for the methodological and evaluation content of later parts of this book.

The opening chapter by McCloskey et al. is a conceptual work by a team of 16 nurses representing health care managers, researchers, and educators. The chapter challenges the traditional description of an "innovation" as pertaining solely to clinical interventions and technologies. It then provides examples of management interventions and the application of systematic evaluation to test the effectiveness of such interventions.

Chapter 2, another conceptually based work, is by Maas, Johnson, and Kraus, members of a research team currently funded to develop and test a classification system for nursing-sensitive patient/client outcomes. This chapter provides brief overviews of the history of outcomes measurement and of the team's research project. Examples of the project, the issues involved in outcomes classification, and the implications for managers are discussed.

Chapter 3, by Courtney, offers insights into the challenges nurse managers will face as health care systems reform forces a transition from hospital-based care to community-based primary care. This is a vital chapter for readers searching for the opportunities this transition creates for professional nurses.

Another transition is addressed by Androwich and Haas (Chapter 4) as they explore outcomes measurement in the rapidly evolving ambulatory health care setting. The unique characteristics of the settings and interventions provided are discussed in terms of the opportunities and challenges offered to nursing.

In the final chapter of Part 1, Ramler, Kraus, Specht, and Titler offer an in-depth description of an internationally used outcomes measurement instrument developed for the Medical Outcomes Studies (MOS). This interpretation of the SF-36 is of special value because it focuses on applications in nursing to measure outcomes at the individual and aggregate client level.

CHAPTER 1

Nursing Management Innovations: A Need for Systematic Evaluation

Joanne Comi McCloskey

Meridean L. Maas

Diane Gardner Huber

Ann Kasparek

Janet Pringle Specht

Cheryl L. Ramler

Carol Watson

Mary A. Blegen

Connie Delaney

Suellyn Ellerbe

Carlie Etscheidt

Carole Gongaware

Marion R. Johnson

Kathleen C. Kelly

Peg Mehmert

Jennifer Clougherty

Nursing research has focused on clinical interventions, with little attention to the equally important management interventions. The concept of management intervention or innovation is introduced here, and five types of management innovations in nursing are identified. An overview of the research base for four of the innovations demonstrates the need for systematic evaluation.

The word *innovations* suggests new technology; however, it also includes new social and organizational ideas. Desired outcomes of new technologies do not happen unless social and organizational innovations keep pace (Kanter, 1983). Although there have been many innovations in biotechnical

AUTHORS' NOTE: This chapter is reprinted with permission of Jannetti Publications, Inc., publisher, *Nursing Economic$*, Volume 12/Number 1 (January/February 1994), pp. 35-44.

knowledge that benefit patient care, equally important management innovations receive little attention.

In response to rapid and sweeping changes in health care technology and resource scarcity, and as a means to improve quality and lower costs, nurse administrators have implemented many organizational and management changes. Few of these have been evaluated systematically for their impact on quality and cost. The mode is to adopt rapidly whatever is "new" or available to meet a pressing need. Management innovations must be evaluated as rigorously as patient care innovations. Current decisions about the effects of management innovations are based on limited data of poor scientific quality. Lacking sound evaluation of their management innovations, managers increase their risk in decision making and may ultimately increase health care costs by implementing organizational changes that are unsound and costly.

The purpose of this chapter is to introduce the idea of nursing management innovations, summarize the research related to four such innovations, and propose a method for more systematic evaluation of these innovations. Viewing management interventions as innovations will assist the nursing management and research communities in understanding better the importance of conducting and funding evaluation research of management innovations.

INNOVATION DEFINED

Innovation is the use of a new idea to solve a problem (Kanter, 1983). According to Drucker (1985), an innovation is the means by which change is exploited as an opportunity for a different business or a different service. Drucker stated that a successful innovation is organized and purposeful, uses knowledge that is already available, does something different, and is simple to understand. Romano (1990b) discussed the difference between change and innovation: Change is disruption, whereas innovation is the use of change to provide new services. For Romano, moving a new idea to the level of innovation requires three things: information, enthusiasm, and authority. The adoption of a new idea or innovation is referred to in much of the literature as *diffusion of innovations,* after the 1983 book with the same title by Everett Rogers. Whereas the general literature on innovations and how they are adopted is fairly large and still growing, the literature on evaluation of innovations is small. In Rogers' terms, innovations create consequences, "the changes that occur to an individual or to a social system as a result of the adoption or rejection of an innovation" (p. 410). Rogers stated that the consequences of innovations have received little attention from change agents or researchers, partially because the methods and measures are difficult. Within health care, there is little research on any aspect of innovations (Sondik, 1989).

Within nursing, research has focused on the study of how new ideas are transferred into practice (Brett, 1989; Johnson, 1990; Ketefian, 1975; Kirchhoff, 1982; Neidlinger, Bartleson, Drews, & Hukari, 1992; Romano, 1990a). There is a good deal of research on the impact of specific personnel attitudes (e.g., job satisfaction, organizational climate), and, in some areas, there are enough studies surrounding clinical innovations to conduct meta-analyses (Devine & Cook, 1983, 1986; Goode et al., 1991; Hathaway, 1986; Schwartz, Mood, Yarandi, & Anderson, 1987). The systematic conceptualization and study of nursing management innovations, however, are lacking.

MANAGEMENT INNOVATIONS

Management innovations are new strategies, structures, or processes for the organization, delivery, and financing of quality care. In nursing, they are implemented at the organizational, departmental, divisional, or unit level. We have identified five types of managerial innovations in nursing: introduction of new technology, personnel development, changes in the organization of work, changes in rewards and incentives, and implementation of quality improvement mechanisms (see Table 1.1). Examples of specific nursing management innovations for each type are identified in the table.

Although many nursing administrators are implementing innovations to enhance service and contain costs, there is currently no systematic method for evaluating their cost-effectiveness. The difficulties with evaluation of the impact of the innovations represent a state-of-the-science deficit rather than poor managerial planning. Given the vast health management literature and the lack of resources and time, health care administrators often must risk changes and decide upon their effectiveness with limited data.

Examples

Four management innovations are presented to illustrate the issues and need for more systematic evaluation. Each of the four innovations represents changes in the organization of work (Category 3 of Table 1.1), a frequent type of management innovation today.

Example 1: Nurse Extenders

Description. The use of nurse extenders is a management innovation aimed at redesigning the care delivery system to achieve the most efficient and cost-

TABLE 1.1 Categories of Nursing Management Innovations, With Examples

1. Introduction of New Technology
     Bedside computers
     Bedside glucose monitors
     Computerized nursing care plan
     Infusion devices
     Nursing information systems

2. Personnel Development
     Certification
     Cross-training/orientation
     Leadership education for nurse managers
     Preceptor programs

3. Changes in Organization of Work
     Case management
     Critical paths/care maps
     Collaborative practice
     Contracted services
     Differentiated practice
     Flexible scheduling
     Nurse extenders/partners in practice
     Product-line management
     Self-scheduling
     Shared governance

4. Changes in Rewards and Incentives
     Clinical ladders/administrative ladders
     Fee for service
     Incentive pay
     Performance recognition programs

5. Implementation of Quality Improvement Mechanisms
     Competency testing
     Peer review
     Quality assurance program
     Technology/product evaluation
     TQM/CQI

effective skill mix of nursing personnel without compromising quality. Unlicensed personnel are added to the nursing staff, with a subsequent increase in the patient-to-RN ratio. Such restructuring is often triggered by the rapidly accelerating pressures to reduce health care costs (Bostrom & Zimmerman, 1993), resulting in experimentation with changed configurations of staff mix and the roles and functions of each category of worker in nursing (Gardner, 1991). The Tri-Council for Nursing's Statement on Assistive Personnel to the Registered Nurse (1990) affirmed that unlicensed personnel historically have assisted RNs in delivering patient care. Ehrat (1990) noted that historically health care organizations have used substitution labor to meet patient care needs because of nurses' failure to define or capitalize on their special contribution to patient outcomes.

Research and Evaluation. Hinshaw (1989) identified the staffing and scheduling of nursing personnel as a major area of nursing administration research. Classic studies on the use of various types of nursing personnel were done by Aydelotte and Tener (1960) and New, Nite, and Callahan (1959). A number of studies have investigated the value and cost of an all-RN staff, concluding that it is less costly and produces more positive staff and patient outcomes (Hartz et al., 1989; Hinshaw, Chance, & Atwood, 1981; Minyard, Wall, & Turner, 1986). Another rich research stream includes the studies evaluating and testing primary nursing (Daeffler, 1975; Flood & Diers, 1988; Gardner & Tilbury, 1991; Giovannetti, 1986; Ventura, Fox, Corley, & Mercurio, 1982; Wolf, Lesic, & Leak, 1986). Giovannetti (1986), however, suggested that the research on primary nursing and desired outcomes is "equivocal." Mallison (1992) suggested linking the results of the *American Journal of Nursing* survey, designed to identify new roles and types of nurse assistants (Blegen, Gardner, & McCloskey, 1992), with studies showing that primary nursing saves money while boosting quality.

Other studies have looked at staffing and scheduling (Flood & Diers, 1988; Fosbinder, 1986; Marchette & Hollomon, 1986; Meiners & Coffey, 1985; Prescott, Dennis, Creasia, & Bowen, 1985; Sovie, Tarcinale, VanPutee, & Stunden, 1985). These studies are diverse, with little replication, and are done in single institutions. Hinshaw (1989) noted that they are difficult to generalize in terms of setting or sample. Few test the effect of nursing staff mix or levels on patient and staff outcomes.

Some evaluation research has been done to identify core nursing tasks and the associated costs of various skill mix ratios (Byrnes, 1982; Davis, 1982; Glandon, Colbert, & Thomasma, 1989; Hamm-Vida, 1990; Hendrickson, Doddato, & Kovner, 1990; Marquess & Petit, 1987). Bostrom and Zimmerman (1993) noted that evaluation of nurse extender programs has been extremely limited. The results of their study showed an impact on the distribution of work and on costs, but no evidence that patient satisfaction or the quality of care improved. No studies were found that used an experimental design or that measured multiple and possibly colinear variables across the range of organizational and patient outcomes to evaluate this innovation. Recent reports either chronicle a case study or describe sparse evaluative efforts related to improved documentation, labor cost savings, or patient satisfaction (Bostrom

& Zimmerman, 1993; Ericksen et al., 1992; O'Brien & Stepura, 1992). In summary, the evaluation of this innovation does not build on prior research and is not of adequate rigor to assert that using nurse extenders is justified for cost, satisfaction, or quality.

Example 2: Hospital-Based Case Management

Description. Case management is a system of "health assessment, planning, procurement, delivery, coordination of services, and monitoring to assure that the multiple service needs of clients are met" (Fuszard et al., 1988, p. 1). Specifically, hospital-based case management is a care delivery system designed for the management of cost and quality outcomes in which an individual, most often a nurse, is responsible for coordinating patient care throughout an episode of illness and across settings (Kramer, 1990; Kruger, 1989; Westhoff, 1992; Zander, 1988a, 1990).

Although conceptually similar to primary nursing, hospital-based case management differs by being more deliberative in planning for resource use and in involving interdisciplinary collaboration. It assumes that length of stay and resource use are costs that can be controlled through more effective timing, sequencing, and coordination of interdisciplinary practice patterns (Williams, 1991; Zander, 1988a). It further assumes that quality can be improved by better understanding and controlling the care delivery process and by standardizing patient, caregiver, and system outcomes (Olivas, Del Togno-Armanasco, Erickson, & Harter, 1989a). In contrast to primary nursing, hospital-based case management emphasizes care management for a larger patient group and increases the use of different levels of direct care providers. It does not expect that all RNs must function as case managers, nor does it assume that all patients must be case managed. Instead, it gives priority to the care management of the chronically ill, high-risk, complicated, or unpredictable patient who does not or cannot adhere to a standardized protocol for care (Kramer, 1990; Kruger, 1989).

The case management model most frequently cited in the literature and most often used as a guide for acute care institutions is the model developed by the New England Medical Center (Zander, 1990). However, a variety of other models with differences in basic concept or application can be found in the literature (Brockopp, Porter, Kinnard, & Silberman, 1992; Cohen, 1991; Fuszard et al., 1988; Marr & Reid, 1992; Schull, Tosch, & Wood, 1992; Stillwaggon, 1989; Westhoff, 1992). Concepts common to all models include (a) cases managed for an episode of illness, (b) accountability for financial and quality outcomes resting with the case manager, (c) interdisciplinary collaboration, and (d) increased patient and family involvement. In addition, most models include one or more of the following: (a) differentiation of the RN role into professional case manager and unit staff nurse; (b) implementation of time-sequenced guidelines for care and anticipated outcomes (critical paths, care maps, protocols, or management action plans); (c) establishment of RN-physician group practices; (d) analysis of individual and aggregate variations in care; and (e) staff education regarding financial aspects of care, communication, and collaboration.

Research and Evaluation. In the literature, case management is generally viewed as an extension of the primary nursing concept or an expansion of the primary nurse's role (Manthey, 1990; Zander, 1990). It has been demonstrated that primary nursing can positively influence health care costs and outcomes (Daeffler, 1975; Gardner & Tilbury, 1991; Giovannetti, 1986; Wolf et al., 1986). Another area of research related to case management is the intensity of nursing care, one of the resources that can be variably allocated or controlled by the case manager. A limited number of studies have noted an association between increased nursing intensity and decreased length of stay (Berki, Ashcroft, & Newbrander, 1984; Halloran & Halloran, 1985; Halloran & Kiley, 1986).

Case management was originally designed in an effort to contain health care costs while maintaining or improving patient outcomes. It is not surprising, then, that cost and patient care outcomes have been emphasized in evaluating this innovation. The financial impact of case management, however, has certainly received the greatest amount of attention in the literature. Financially, case-managed and non-case-managed patient populations have been compared in regard to average length of stay, cost per case, charge per case, and reimbursement per case (Bair, Griswold, & Head, 1989; Brockopp et al., 1992; Cohen, 1991; Ethridge & Lamb, 1989; Marr & Reid, 1992; McKenzie, Torkelson, & Holt, 1989; Olivas, Del Togno-Armanasco, Erickson, & Harter, 1989b; Schull et al., 1992; Sinnen & Schifalacqua, 1991; Smith, Massicotte Pass, Pounovich-Stream, & Jones, 1993; Weber, 1992; Zander, 1988b). Calculation of costs, charges, and reimbursement varies among studies. Reduced costs are due to shortening the length of stay, but direct care time during the stay increases (Cohen, 1991), and focusing only on hospital costs may mask cost shifts to other parts of the health care system. Only one study (Cohen, 1991) has attempted to determine statistical significance of the data.

With regard to patient care outcomes, the research has varied. With the exception of patient satisfaction, there is little consistency in the selection of the outcome measures. Patient satisfaction is most often reported anecdotally or from information returned on hospital-specific satisfaction surveys (Brockopp et al., 1992; McKenzie et al., 1989; Millinson, 1988; Olivas et al., 1989b; Schull et al., 1992; Sinnen & Schifalacqua, 1991; Smith et al., 1993; Stillwaggon, 1989; Zander, 1988b). No standard patient satisfaction survey tools were reported as being used. Nurse satisfaction and physician satisfaction were noted only anecdotally in three articles (Brockopp et al., 1992; Olivas et al., 1989b; Weber, 1992). In summary, case management is being implemented in many hospitals, mainly in attempts to reduce health care costs. Little research is available to demonstrate cost- or quality effectiveness.

Example 3: Nursing Shared Governance

Description. An organization's authority ordinarily is vested in positions, with those positions higher in the hierarchy assigned a greater scope of authority. *Nursing shared governance* refers to shared authority and accountability for decision making by nurses and the organization to meet the mandates of the profession and the goals of the organization (Maas & Specht, 1994; Porter-O'Grady, 1991). Shared governance is an organizational structure for decision making, formalized with bylaws and implemented through processes for nurse participation (e.g., standard setting, peer review). Although models vary greatly, there is consensus that nursing shared governance means that professional nursing staff autonomy is increased and that decision making is shared by nursing professionals and nursing management. There is less agreement regarding the scope of nursing staff autonomy—for example, what decisions should be retained by nurse managers and how nursing staff should be included in the governance structures (Maas & Specht, 1994).

   Although there have been isolated examples of implementation over several decades (Horvath, 1990; Jacoby & Terpstra, 1990; Johnson, 1987; Jones & Ortiz, 1989; Maas & Jacox, 1977; McDonagh, Rhodes, Sharkey, & Goodroe, 1989; Rose & DiPasquale, 1990), examples of nursing shared governance in hospitals have been more frequent since the 1980s. Reasons given in the literature to implement shared governance in nursing include facilitating professional nurse autonomy and job satisfaction, enhancing organizational effectiveness, and achieving quality patient outcomes.

Research and Evaluation of Nursing Shared Governance. A variety of models have been reported that purport to enable nurse autonomy in employing organizations, yet descriptions of specific structures and processes and how these enable nurse autonomy are often lacking. Most reports of the effects of shared governance models are anecdotal, focusing on effects on nurses' perceived autonomy and job satisfaction. Few studies have examined the relationship between nurse decision-making autonomy and the achievement of quality patient outcomes (Batey & Lewis, 1982; Knaus, Draper, Wagner, & Zimmerman, 1986). Evaluation of shared governance is difficult due to the complexity of the concept, the variety of definitions, and the frequent implementation in conjunction with other nursing management and practice innovations, such as case management.

Alexander, Weisman, and Chase (1982) found that nurses' perceived autonomy was higher on units that used primary nursing and had lower workloads. However, McCloskey (1990) found that perceived autonomy was not clearly related to workload and noted that several organizational variables may influence nurses' perceptions of autonomy. Several studies have found that nurses' perceived autonomy is a major explanatory variable in job satisfaction (McCloskey, 1990; Munro, 1983; Roedel & Nystrom, 1988; Seybolt, 1986; Slavitt, Stamps, Piedmont, & Haase, 1978). Pinkerton (1988) and Ludemann and Brown (1989) evaluated the effects of implementation of nursing shared governance models, and Ethridge (1987) tested the effects of multiple organizational changes, including shared governance and a case management system. It is difficult to evaluate these studies because they did not clearly define their organizational structures. Perceived autonomy was used as the measure of nurse autonomy.

Finally, although research on nurse autonomy emphasizes the influence of organizational structures and processes on autonomy, these features tend to be addressed together, thereby masking the effects of any one feature. There is a lack of standardization of shared governance models, and the specific structures and processes that are implemented are usually not clearly specified. Measurement of actual decisions in matters other than clinical practice that affect nursing practice, measurement of authority for decisions by nursing staff as a collective, and measurement of patient outcome effects of nursing shared governance are largely neglected. Adequate longitudinal and multisite data are lacking due to the complexity and cost of the research. Thus studies to evaluate shared governance tend to lack rigor, yield mixed results, leave questions as to what has been evaluated, and produce little opportunity for comparing results.

Example 4: Product-Line Management

Description. This innovation is not unique to health care. It was originally adopted in industry in the early 1960s (Folger & Gee, 1987). *Product-line management* refers to the management of resources used in the creation of a given product (Porter-O'Grady, 1989). The product is defined as the outcome of the work of the organization or a subset of the organization. In health care, examples are home health care, cancer care, and maternity care.

Instituting product-line management requires a decentralized organizational structure rather than the traditional hierarchy (Flynn, 1991; Murray, 1989). A matrix type of organization is needed to facilitate both horizontal and vertical coordination of services and decision making. Decisions must be made close to the "point of action," with those in control of production empowered to accomplish the outcomes. Philosophically, product-line management broadens the focus of care from quality only to cost and productivity, requiring that the clinical manager have strong financial and management skills.

A similar concept, *service-line management,* refers to a collection of like services coordinated by an organizational structure that facilitates client needs throughout the service delivery (Bruhn & Howes, 1986; Porter-O'Grady, 1989). The focus of service-line management, in contrast to the cost/productivity focus of product-line management, is on the planning/management system for individual clients. However, many of the same characteristics, such as decentralized decision making, matrix structure, and marketing, are used in both, and often the terms are used interchangeably.

Research and Evaluation. The evaluation of the effectiveness of product-line management has been limited. Although information defining product-line management and extolling its merits abounds, research is limited to case descriptions. Because it is a change at the organizational level, sample size and comparisons are difficult. Case studies in nursing (Fackelmann, 1985; Montgomery, 1989; Murray, 1989; Vosburgh, 1991) illustrate some of the difficulties of implementation. Although the studies discuss financial outcomes, the impact on quality of care and job design is neglected. Individual components of product-line management have been described (Flarey, 1991; Stanton, 1986), but attempts to evaluate the implementation of the total redesign of the organizational structure and philosophy are limited. Thus there is essentially no research to document the advantages or disadvantages of an innovation that took the hospital community by storm in the 1980s and is now dying out.

Summary

These examples illustrate common difficulties encountered with research to evaluate nursing management innovations (see Table 1.2). The innovations are

TABLE 1.2 Difficulties Encountered With Research to Evaluate Nursing
           Management Innovations

---

1. Complex innovations lack clear definitions.
2. Innovations are often implemented with other changes, making it difficult to isolate the effect.
3. The group level of measurement makes it difficult to obtain large samples.
4. The intervening variables are not often identified, controlled for, or measured.
5. The effects on staff and patients tend to be ignored.

---

usually complex, often lack clear definition, and tend to be introduced along with other organizational and practice changes. Whether they are implemented at the unit, division, or organization level, it is difficult to obtain large sample sizes. Typically, studies are site specific, are not based on the results of prior research, and do not employ experimental designs with sufficient controls to identify the effect of the innovation. Multisite, longitudinal studies are very difficult and costly to implement due to lack of standardization of the innovations, the complexity of the innovations, and the diversity of sites. Although costs of the innovations are often examined, staff and patient outcomes tend to be ignored. In general, results cannot be compared across sites because of lack of standardization of the innovations and the outcomes that are measured.

A PROPOSED SOLUTION

Systematic evaluation strategies for more effective and efficient management of nursing services are central to improving health care and reducing costs. At the University of Iowa, a "suitcase methodology" was invented to evaluate the impact of management innovations. A set of variables and their measures that could be used to assist organizations to evaluate management innovations were identified. The goal of this project was to provide a "readiness for research" evaluation system that could be implemented quickly when organizations put innovations in place. To date, research instruments and information on over 300 instruments helpful to the evaluation of management innovations have been collected. Each instrument is being systematically evaluated for its psychometric properties and its ease of use. Developing a suitcase or portfolio of usable instruments for evaluating management innovations is essential. When executives know that an innovation is about to be implemented, they can use the suitcase methodology for assistance with measurement, design, and instru-

TABLE 1.3   Types of Variables to Measure in Evaluation of Organizational Change

1. *Personnel*—the attitudes and work of nurses and their assistants (e.g., job satisfaction, autonomy, organizational commitment, social integration, professionalism, motivation, conflict, job performance)

2. *Organizational*—the nature of the organization (e.g., organizational climate, decentralization, innovation, routinization, turnover, absenteeism, leadership style)

3. *Patient Outcomes*—results of health care interventions as perceived/experienced by the recipient of the intervention (e.g., functional status, general well-being, satisfaction with care, changes in signs and symptoms)

4. *Cost*—Costs of implementation (e.g., personnel time, equipment, training costs)

5. *Demographics*—on the nurses (e.g., education, experience, age), the organization (e.g., type of unit, delivery of care method, staff mix), and the patients (e.g., age, medical diagnoses, nursing diagnoses, length of treatment)

ments. An evaluation package would be prescribed on the basis of the nature of their innovation and the desired change.

Any evaluation of an organizational innovation must consider five types of variables: personnel, organizational, patient outcomes, cost, and demographics (see Table 1.3). The appropriate variables for measurement would be identified on the basis of the answers to the set of questions listed in Table 1.4. Using a standardized measurement of these variables will help determine the effect of any changes. With so many changes happening so fast, it is not possible to design a separate study to examine every change. If standardized data were

TABLE 1.4   Guidelines for Selecting the Variables to Measure in Order to
Demonstrate the Impact of a Management Innovation

1. Describe the innovation.

2. What is the desired outcome? What is motivating the innovation?

3. At what level of the organization is the change you wish to measure?

4. Who will be affected by the innovation (e.g., organization, staff, patients, family)? To what extent and in what way will they be affected?

5. What does the research about the innovation demonstrate: That is, what results are known usually to happen?

6. What else is going on in the organization at the same time that might mediate the effects of the innovation?

7. When do results need to be demonstrated?

8. Are there any natural mechanisms (e.g., regular meetings, evaluation conferences, clinic visits) for collecting data that could be used?

9. What measures are already available? Are these in easily usable form?

collected at regular intervals on, say, unit and organization demographics and staff satisfaction, commitment and intent to stay, and patient satisfaction and specific functional health status indicators, the effectiveness of new innovations could be determined. Every nurse in the health care agency should complete a short battery of instruments on a regular basis (every 6 months). In addition, patient outcomes data should be collected in a routine manner. This will generate baseline data for any organization change.

Please note that currently these are ideas only. We are not yet able to provide this kind of assistance and do not in fact know if it will work. These ideas are offered to assist nurse executives who are faced daily with the need for evaluation. The rapid changes of the health care system in response to the needs of patients, health care advances, and resource constraints will continue to require quick implementation of management innovations. The evaluation of the effectiveness of these innovations is essential for several reasons: (a) A large portion of any health care institution's budget is in the nursing department, (b) nearly all health care innovations in health care institutions involve and influence nursing staff, (c) the retention and performance of nurses are very important in the delivery of quality patient care, and (d) methods to evaluate the impact of health care innovations in which nurses play a key role have been neglected. The costly U.S. health care system cannot afford *not* to invest in the evaluation of nursing management innovations.

REFERENCES

Alexander, C. S., Weisman, C. S., & Chase, G. A. (1982). Determinants of staff nurses' perceptions of autonomy within different clinical contexts. *Nursing Research, 31*(1), 48-52.

Aydelotte, M. K., & Tener, M. (1960). *An investigation of the relation between nursing activity and patient welfare.* Iowa City: University of Iowa.

Bair, N. L., Griswold, J. T., & Head, J. L. (1989). Clinical RN involvement in bedside-centered case management. *Nursing Economic$, 7*(3), 150-154.

Batey, M. V., & Lewis, F. M. (1982). Clarifying autonomy and accountability in nursing service: Part 1. *Journal of Nursing Administration, 12*(9), 13-18.

Berki, S. E., Ashcroft, M. L., & Newbrander, W. C. (1984). Length of stay variations within ICDA-8 diagnosis related groups. *Medical Care, 22,* 126.

Blegen, M., Gardner, D., & McCloskey, J. (1992). Survey results: Who helps you with your work? *American Journal of Nursing, 92*(1), 26-31.

Bostrom, J., & Zimmerman, J. (1993). Restructuring nursing for a competitive health care environment. *Nursing Economic$, 11*(1), 35-41, 54.

Brett, J. (1989). Organizational integrative mechanisms and adoption of innovations by nurses. *Nursing Research, 38*(2), 105-110.

Brockopp, D. Y., Porter, M., Kinnard, S., & Silberman, S. (1992). Fiscal and clinical evaluation of patient care: A case management model for the future. *Journal of Nursing Administration, 22*(9), 23-27.

Bruhn, P. S., & Howes, D. H. (1986). Service line management: New opportunities for nursing executives. *Journal of Nursing Administration, 16*(6), 13-18.

Byrnes, M. (1982). Non-nursing functions: The nurses state their case. *American Journal of Nursing, 82,* 1089-1092.

Cohen, E. L. (1991). Nursing case management: Does it pay? *Journal of Nursing Administration, 21*(4), 20-25.

Daeffler, R. (1975). Patients' perceptions of care under team and primary nursing. *Journal of Nursing Administration, 5*(3), 20-26.

Davis, K. (1982). Non-nursing functions: Our readers respond. *American Journal of Nursing, 82,* 1857-1860.

Devine, E. C., & Cook, T. D. (1983). A meta-analysis of effects of psychoeducational interventions on length of post surgical hospital stay. *Nursing Research, 33,* 267-274.

Devine, E. C., & Cook, T. D. (1986). Clinical and cost saving effects of psychoeducational interventions with surgical patients: A meta-analysis. *Research in Nursing and Health, 9,* 89-105.

Drucker, P. F. (1985). *Innovation and entrepreneurship: Practice and principles.* New York: Harper & Row.

Ehrat, K. (1990). *Administrative issues and approaches.* Chicago: American Hospital Association.

Ericksen, L., Quandt, B., Teinert, D., Look, D., Loosle, R., Mackey, G., & Strout, B. (1992). A registered nurse-licensed vocational nurse partnership model for critical care nursing. *Journal of Nursing Administration, 22*(12), 28-38.

Ethridge, P. (1987). Nurse accountability program improves satisfaction, turnover. *Health Progress, 68*(5), 44-49.

Ethridge, P., & Lamb, G. S. (1989). Professional nursing case management improves quality, access, and costs. *Nursing Management, 20*(3), 30-35.

Fackelmann, K. A. (1985, November 22). Cleveland hospital on the road to product line management. *Modern Healthcare,* pp. 70-77.

Flarey, D. L. (1991). Redesigning management roles: The executive challenge. *Journal of Nursing Administration, 21*(2), 40-45.

Flood, S., & Diers, D. (1988). Nurse staffing, patient outcome and cost. *Nursing Management, 19*(5), 34-43.

Flynn, M. K. (1991). Product-line management: Threat or opportunity for nursing? *Nursing Administration Quarterly, 15*(2), 21-32.

Folger, J. C., & Gee, E. P. (1987). *Product management for hospitals: Organizing for profitability.* Chicago: American Hospital Publishing.

Fosbinder, D. (1986). Nursing costs/DRG: A patient classification system and comparative study. *Journal of Nursing Administration, 16,* 18-23.

Fuszard, B., Bowman, R., Howell, H. T., Malinoski, A., Morrison, C., & Wahlstedt, P. (1988). *Nursing case management.* Kansas City, MO: American Nurses Association.

Gardner, D. (1991). Issues related to the use of nurse extenders. *Journal of Nursing Administration, 21*(10), 40-45.

Gardner, K., & Tilbury, M. (1991). A longitudinal cost analysis of primary and team nursing. *Nursing Economic$, 9*(2), 97-104.

Giovannetti, P. (1986). Evaluation of primary nursing. *Annual Review of Nursing Research, 4,* 127-152.

Glandon, G., Colbert, K., & Thomasma, M. (1989). Nursing delivery models and RN mix: Cost implications. *Nursing Management, 20*(5), 30-33.

Goode, C. J., Titler, M., Rakel, B., Ones, D., Kleiber, C., Small, S., & Triolo, P. (1991). A meta-analysis of effects of heparin flush and saline flush: Quality and cost implications. *Nursing Research, 40,* 321-330.

Halloran, E., & Halloran, D. (1985). Exploring the DRG/nursing equation. *American Journal of Nursing, 85,* 1093-1095.

Halloran, E., & Kiley, M. (1986). Case mix management. *Nursing Management, 15*, 39-45.

Hamm-Vida, D. (1990). Cost of non-nursing tasks. *Nursing Management, 21*(4), 46-52.

Hartz, A., Krakauer, M., Kuhn, E., Young, M., Jacobsen, S., Gay, G., Muenz, L., Katzoff, M., Bailey, R., & Rimm, A. (1989). Hospital characteristics and mortality rates. *New England Journal of Medicine, 321*, 1720-1725.

Hathaway, D. (1986). Effect of preoperative instruction on postoperative outcomes: A meta-analysis. *Nursing Research, 35*, 269-275.

Hendrickson, G., Doddato, T., & Kovner, C. (1990). How do nurses use their time? *Journal of Nursing Administration, 20*(3), 31-37.

Hinshaw, A. (1989). Programs of nursing research for nursing administration. In B. Henry, C. Arndt, M. DiVincenti, & A. Marriner-Tomey (Eds.), *Dimensions of nursing administration: Theory, research, education, practice* (pp. 251-266). Boston: Blackwell.

Hinshaw, A., Chance, H., & Atwood, J. (1981). Staff, patient and cost outcomes of all-registered nurse staffing. *Journal of Nursing Administration, 11*(11-12), 30-36.

Horvath, K. J. (1990). Professional nursing practice model. In G. G. Mayer, M. J. Madden, & E. Lawrenz (Eds.), *Patient care delivery models* (pp. 213-235). Rockville, MD: Aspen.

Jacoby, J., & Terpstra, M. (1990). Collaborative governance: Model for professional autonomy. *Nursing Management, 21*(2), 42-44.

Johnson, L. M. (1987). Self-governance: Treatment for an unhealthy nursing culture. *Health Progress, 68*(5), 41-43.

Johnson, M. B. (1990). The holistic paradigm in nursing: The diffusion of an innovation. *Research in Nursing and Health, 13*, 129-139.

Jones, L. S., & Ortiz, M. E. (1989). Increasing nurse autonomy and recognition through shared governance. *Nursing Administration Quarterly, 13*(4), 11-16.

Kanter, R. M. (1983). *The change masters: Innovation for productivity in the American corporation.* New York: Simon & Schuster.

Ketefian, S. (1975). Application of selected nursing research findings into nursing practice. *Nursing Research, 24*, 89-92.

Kirchhoff, K. T. (1982). A diffusion survey of coronary precautions. *Nursing Research, 31*, 196-201.

Knaus, W., Draper, E., Wagner, D., & Zimmerman, J. (1986). An evaluation of outcome from intensive care in major medical centers. *Annals of Internal Medicine, 104*, 410-418.

Kramer, M. (1990). The magnet hospitals: Excellence revisited. *Journal of Nursing Administration, 20*(9), 39-40.

Kruger, N. R. (1989). Case management: Is it a delivery system for my organization? *Aspen Advisor for Nurse Executives, 4*(10), 4, 5, 8.

Ludemann, R. S., & Brown, C. (1989). Staff perceptions of shared governance. *Nursing Administration Quarterly, 13*(4), 49-56.

Maas, M. L., & Jacox, A. K. (1977). *Guidelines for nurse autonomy/patient welfare.* New York: Appleton-Century-Crofts.

Maas, M. L., & Specht, J. P. (1994). Shared governance in nursing: What is shared, who governs, and who benefits? In J. McCloskey & H. Grace (Eds.), *Current issues in nursing* (4th ed., pp. 398-406). St. Louis: C. V. Mosby.

Mallison, M. (1992). Look under the hood. *American Journal of Nursing, 92*, 7.

Manthey, M. (1990). Definitions and basic elements of a patient care delivery system with an emphasis on primary nursing. In G. G. Mayer, M. J. Madden, & E. Lawrenz (Eds.), *Patient care delivery models* (pp. 201-212). Rockville, MD: Aspen.

Marchette, L., & Hollomon, F. (1986). Length of stay: Significant variables. *Journal of Nursing Administration, 16*, 12-19.

Marquess, R., & Petit, B. (1987). An analysis of the effects of percent RN staff on nursing costs by DRG. *Nursing Management, 18*(5), 33-36.

Marr, J., & Reid, B. (1992). Implementing managed care and case management: The neuroscience experience. *Journal of Neuroscience Nursing, 24*(5), 281-285.

McCloskey, J. C. (1990). Two requirements for job contentment: Autonomy and social integration. *Image, 22,* 140-143.

McDonagh, K. J., Rhodes, B., Sharkey, K., & Goodroe, J. H. (1989). Shared governance at Saint Joseph's Hospital of Atlanta: A mature professional practice model. *Nursing Administration Quarterly, 13*(4), 17-28.

McKenzie, C. B., Torkelson, N. G., & Holt, M. A. (1989). Care and cost: Nursing case management improves both. *Nursing Management, 20*(10), 30-34.

Meiners, M., & Coffey, R. (1985). Hospital DRGs and the need for long-term care services: An empirical analysis. *Health Services Research, 20,* 360-384.

Millinson, M. (1988, September 17). Nursing case management: A success at Boston Hospital. *Health Week,* p. 31.

Minyard, K., Wall, J., & Turner, R. (1986). RNs may cost less than you think. *Journal of Nursing Administration, 16*(5), 28-34.

Montgomery, S. K. (1989). A case study implementation of strategic business units. In M. Johnson (Ed.), *Series on nursing administration: Vol. 2. Changing organizational structure* (pp. 23-41). Redwood, CA: Addison-Wesley.

Munro, B. H. (1983). Job satisfaction among recent graduates of schools of nursing. *Nursing Research, 32,* 350-355.

Murray, K. G. (1989). Program administration: A product line approach. In M. Johnson (Ed.), *Series on nursing administration: Vol. 2. Changing organizational structure* (pp. 44-66). Redwood, CA: Addison-Wesley.

Neidlinger, S. H., Bartleson, B. H., Drews, N., & Hukari, D. (1992). Venture actualization in nursing: An analysis of innovation. *Journal of Nursing Administration, 22*(7/8), 65-70.

New, P., Nite, G., & Callahan, J. (1959, October). Too many nurses may be worse than too few. *Modern Hospital,* pp. 104-106.

O'Brien, Y., & Stepura, B. (1992). Designing roles for assistive personnel in a rural hospital. *Journal of Nursing Administration, 22*(10), 34-37.

Olivas, G. S., Del Togno-Armanasco, V., Erickson, J. R., & Harter, S. (1989a). Case management: A bottom-line care delivery model—Part 1: The concept. *Journal of Nursing Administration, 19*(11), 16-20.

Olivas, G. S., Del Tongo-Armanasco, V., Erickson, J. R., & Harter, S. (1989b). Case management: A bottom-line care delivery model—Part 2: Adaptation of the model. *Journal of Nursing Administration, 19*(12), 12-17.

Pinkerton, S. (1988). Evaluation of shared governance in a nursing department. In M. Stull & S. Pinkerton (Eds.), *Current strategies for nurse administrators* (pp. 141-150). Rockville, MD: Aspen.

Porter-O'Grady, T. (1989). Product-line management for nursing: A new framework for service. In M. Johnson (Ed.), *Series on nursing administration: Vol. 2. Changing organizational structure* (pp. 129-143). Redwood, CA: Addison-Wesley.

Porter-O'Grady, T. (1991). Shared governance for nursing, part 1: Creating the new organization. *AORN Journal, 53,* 458-466.

Prescott, P., Dennis, K., Creasia, J., & Bowen, S. (1985). Nursing shortage in transition. *Image, 18,* 127-133.

Roedel, R. R., & Nystrom, P. C. (1988). Nursing jobs and satisfaction. *Nursing Management, 16,* 34-38.

Rogers, E. M. (1983). *Diffusion of innovations* (3rd ed.). New York: Free Press.

Romano, C. A. (1990a). Diffusion of technology innovation. *Advances in Nursing Science, 13*(2), 11-21.

Romano, C. A. (1990b). Innovation: The promise and the perils for nursing and information technology. *Computers in Nursing, 8*(3), 99-104.

Rose, M., & DiPasquale, B. (1990). The Johns Hopkins professional practice model. In G. G. Mayer, M. J. Madden, & E. Lawrenz (Eds.), *Patient care delivery models* (pp. 85-97). Rockville, MD: Aspen.

Schull, D. E., Tosch, P., & Wood, M. (1992). Clinical nurse specialists as collaborative care managers. *Nursing Management, 23*(3), 38-42.

Schwartz, R., Mood, L., Yarandi, H., & Anderson, G. C. (1987). A meta-analysis of critical outcome variables in nonnutritive sucking in preterm infants. *Nursing Research, 36,* 292-295.

Seybolt, J. W. (1986). Dealing with premature employee turnover. *Journal of Nursing Administration, 16*(2), 64-73.

Sinnen, M. T., & Schifalacqua, M. M. (1991). Coordinated care in a community hospital. *Nursing Management, 22*(3), 30-33.

Slavitt, D. B., Stamps, P. L., Piedmont, E. B., & Haase, A. M. (1978). Nurses' satisfaction with their work situation. *Nursing Research, 27,* 114-120.

Smith, P., Massicotte Pass, C., Pounovich-Stream, C., & Jones, B. (1993). Implementing nurse case management in a community hospital. *MEDSURG Nursing, 1*(11), 47-52.

Sondik, E. J. (1989). Discussion of diffusion of medical innovations. In P. N. Anderson, P. F. Engstrom, & L. E. Mortenson (Eds.), *Advances in cancer control: Innovations and research* (pp. 35-39). New York: Alan R. Liss.

Sovie, M., Tarcinale, M., VanPutee, A., & Stunden, A. (1985). Amalgam of nursing acuity, DRGs and costs. *Nursing Management, 16,* 22-42.

Stanton, L. J. (1986). Nursing care and nursing products: Revenue or expenses. *Journal of Nursing Administration, 16*(9), 29-32.

Stillwaggon, C. (1989). The impact of nurse managed care on the cost of nurse practice and nurse satisfaction. *Journal of Nursing Administration, 12*(11), 21-27.

Tri-Council for Nursing. (1990). *Statement on assistive personnel to the registered nurse.* Washington, DC: American Association of Colleges of Nursing.

Ventura, M., Fox, R., Corley, M., & Mercurio, S. (1982). A patient satisfaction measure as a criterion to evaluate primary nursing. *Nursing Research, 31,* 226-230.

Vosburgh, M. L. (1991). Product-line management through organizational redesign. *Nursing Administration Quarterly, 15*(2), 39-48.

Weber, D. O. (1992). Case study: Clinical pathways stretch patient care but shrink costly lengths of stay at Anne Arundel Medical Center in Annapolis, Maryland. *Strategies for Healthcare Excellence, 5*(5), 1-9.

Westhoff, L. (1992). Care management: Quelling the confusion. *Health Progress, 73,* 43-46, 58.

Williams, B. S. (1991). The utility of nursing theory in nursing case management practice. *Nursing Administration Quarterly, 15*(3), 60-65.

Wolf, G., Lesic, L., & Leak, A. (1986). Primary nursing: The impact of costs within DRGs. *Journal of Nursing Administration, 16*(3), 9-11.

Zander, K. (1988a). Nursing case management: Resolving the DRG paradox. *Nursing Clinics of North America, 23,* 503-520.

Zander, K. (1988b). Nursing case management: Strategic management of cost and quality outcomes. *Journal of Nursing Administration, 18*(5), 23-30.

Zander, K. (1990). Managed care and nursing case management. In G. G. Mayer, M. J. Madden, & E. Lawrenz (Eds.), *Patient care delivery models* (pp. 37-61). Rockville, MD: Aspen.

CHAPTER 2

Nursing-Sensitive Patient Outcomes Classification

Meridean L. Maas
Marion R. Johnson
Vicki L. Kraus

This chapter provides an overview of work by a research team at the University of Iowa College of Nursing to classify nursing-sensitive patient outcomes. A historical review of outcome measurement is highlighted in relation to the current emphasis on patient outcomes. The aims and methods of the project are described briefly. Examples of work in progress are provided. Conceptual issues related to outcome measurement are discussed throughout the chapter, as are implications for nurse administrators.

Concerns about cost, quality, and distribution have fueled a demand for research that demonstrates the effectiveness of nursing management and clinical interventions. These circumstances and the recognized need for standardized languages to enable computerized uniform nursing data sets (Lange & Jacox, 1993; McCloskey & Bulechek, 1994; Werley & Lang, 1988) have

AUTHORS' NOTE: The research reported in this chapter was assisted by grants from Sigma Theta Tau International and the National Center of Nursing Research (NIH 1R01NR03437-01, M. Johnson and M. Maas, Co-Principal Investigators). The following individuals are also members of the research team: Sandra Bellinger, Veronica Brighton, Ginette Budreau, Jeanette Daly, M. Patricia Donahue, Joyce Eland, Deborah Jensen, Kathleen Kelly, Tom Kruckeberg, Ann Lewis, Jeanette Miller, Sue Moorhead, Colleen Prophet, Margaret Rankin, Elizabeth A. Swanson, Bonnie Westra, Marilyn Willits, and George Woodworth.

highlighted the need for a classification of nursing-sensitive patient outcomes. Although classifications of nursing diagnoses (North American Nursing Diagnosis Association [NANDA], 1992; Martin & Scheet, 1992) and nursing interventions (Iowa Intervention Project, 1992; Saba et al., 1991) have been developed, a classification of nursing-sensitive patient outcomes that is useful for multiple purposes, including the evaluation of management interventions, has not yet been accomplished. Nursing's ability to assess its effectiveness is seriously hampered by the lack of a standardized language for patient outcomes influenced by nursing management and clinical interventions. Nurse administrators in particular are handicapped by the lack of standardized outcomes in the development of computerized nursing information systems and in the use of standardized databases to evaluate the effectiveness of management innovations and clinical nursing services.

This chapter provides an overview of work by a research team at the University of Iowa College of Nursing to classify nursing-sensitive patient outcomes. Following a discussion of factors and events that have led to the research, the purposes, aims, and methods for the project are described, including progress in development of the classification and selected examples of outcomes and associated indicators. Conceptual and methodological issues are discussed throughout the chapter, with implications for nurse administrators elaborated in the final section.

HISTORICAL BACKGROUND

The study of patient outcomes began with Florence Nightingale's analysis of health care conditions during the Crimean War (Lang & Marek, 1990; Salive, Mayfield, & Weissman, 1990). Since that time, the measurement of patient outcomes has been sporadic, often discipline specific, and frequently focused on medical practice. Selected major developments in the use of patient outcomes to measure health care quality and effectiveness are outlined in Table 2.1.

In the 1990s, there has been considerable work to develop instruments to measure patient outcomes, such as the SF-36 (see Ramler, Kraus, Specht, & Titler, Chapter 5 of this book). Efforts are also under way to develop generic report cards to measure the effectiveness of health care delivery organizations (Bergman, 1993; Darby, 1993).

Table 2.1 illustrates a number of trends in outcome development. First, nursing has played an active role in the development of outcome criteria relevant to nursing practice. Second, work that has been done outside of nursing has focused on physician practice. Third, the focus of outcome evaluation has changed from an emphasis on efficacy to an emphasis on effective-

TABLE 2.1 Developments in Use of Patient Outcomes for Nursing Effectiveness
           Research

Date	Development
1910	Ernest Codman developed the "End Result System," an outcome-based quality measure, for the evaluation of physician practice (Lembke, 1959).
1962	Myrtle Aydelotte (1962) used patient welfare to evaluate the impact of structural changes in nursing care.
1966	Avedis Donabedian (1966) developed the structure, process, and outcome framework for evaluating the quality of patient care.
1968	The National Center for Health Services Research (NCHSR) was established.
1973	Wennberg and Giltelsohn (1973) reported wide variations in physician practice patterns. The American Nurses Association (ANA) published generic and specialty practice standards.
1977	The ANA (1977) published *Guidelines for Review of Nursing Care at the Local Level*, which included the ANA Model of Quality Assurance, guidelines for developing outcome criteria, and sets of sample standards and outcome criteria.
1978	Hover and Zimmer (1978) developed five categories of nursing-sensitive outcome criteria to be used for quality assurance. Horn and Swain (1978) developed and tested over 500 items to measure the effectiveness of nursing care.
1984	Lang and Clinton (1984) published a review of research measuring the quality of nursing care.
1986	The Patient Outcome Assessment Research Program of the NCHSR was established. The ANA Board of Directors adopted a policy supporting the development of classification systems for nursing diagnoses, nursing interventions, and nursing-sensitive patient outcomes (Lang & Marek, 1990).

ness. Efficacy research tests the outcome effects of interventions under controlled conditions (Lohr, 1988). Effectiveness evaluation measures relative costs and outcomes of different modes of treatment and has focused research on patient outcomes as measures of effectiveness (Ozbolt, 1991).

SIGNIFICANCE

The prominence of patient outcomes in effectiveness research has made the identification of patient outcomes that are sensitive to nursing interventions a major priority (Lower & Burton, 1989; Marek, 1989). Although assessing the effectiveness of medical practice is emphasized, professional nursing, led by the National Center for Nursing Research (NCNR) and the American

TABLE 2.1 *Continued*

Date	Development
1987	The Joint Commission published its Agenda for Change and initiated its clinical indicator project (O'Leary, 1987; Skolnick, 1993).
1988	Kathleen Lohr (1988) published a classic article on outcome measurement, including conceptual and measurement issues.
	The Health Care Financing Administration's (HCFA's) Medical Effectiveness Initiative was launched to improve the quality of medical information available for practice (Roper, Winkenwerder, Hackbarth, & Krakauer, 1988).
1989	Marek (1989) identified 15 outcome categories used to evaluate nursing care.
	The Agency for Health Care Policy and Research (AHCPR) was established, with responsibility for the Medical Effectiveness Treatment Program (MEDTEP). MEDTEP was charged with medical effectiveness treatment research, developing and disseminating practice guidelines, and developing databases (AHCPR, 1990).
	The ANA Congress of Nursing Practice appointed a Task Force on Nursing Practice Standards.
	The Medical Outcomes Study (MOS) used four broad categories to measure the effect of physician structure and process on patient outcomes (Tarlov et al., 1989).
1990	The ANA Congress of Nursing Practice established a Steering Committee on Databases.
1991	The National Center for Nursing Research (NCNR) sponsored a State of the Science Conference, Patient Outcomes Research: Examining the Effectiveness of Nursing Practice.
	The Nursing-Sensitive Outcomes Classification (NOC) research team was formed at the University of Iowa College of Nursing to develop a classification of nursing-sensitive patient outcomes.

Nurses Association (ANA), realized that the focus on effectiveness is a challenge to all health care disciplines (see Table 2.1). An important result of the current emphasis on evaluation of the effectiveness of health care interventions has been the recognition that all initiatives require the identification, standardization, and valid measurement of patient outcomes (McCloskey & Bulechek, 1994).

Advances in computer technology also have contributed to the need for standardized languages by making it feasible to use national data sets for health care evaluation and outcomes research. For example, HCFA collects data on mortality, morbidity, disability, and cost for Medicaid and Medicare recipients and is expanding the database to monitor variations in interventions and outcomes (Roper, 1990). In addition, the federal government is investigating the feasibility of linking clinical, research, and administrative data (AHCPR, 1991). It is clear that the development and use of large data sets will accelerate with technologic advances. Thus it is imperative that nursing develop standardized languages to be represented in national data sets.

The political interest in outcomes, in conjunction with the development and use of national data sets, has put pressure on physicians and others to define and justify what they are about (Brook, 1989) and has created a distinct area of study that Wennberg calls *clinical evaluation science* (DeFriese, 1990). For nursing to become a full participant in this developing discipline, it is essential that patient outcomes influenced by nursing management and clinical interventions be identified and measured (Jennings, 1991; Lower & Burton, 1989; Marek, 1989). Although it is recognized that the majority of patient outcomes, including those traditionally used to evaluate physician care, are not influenced by any one discipline alone, it is important that nursing identify patient outcomes most influenced by nursing care. Nurse managers need this information to direct and evaluate nursing care in their organizations. The profession needs the information to ensure the inclusion of nursing-sensitive outcomes in the evaluation of its services. As Mallison (1990) noted in an *American Journal of Nursing* editorial, if nursing relies on physician-centered information only, "The impact of nursing care will remain largely unmeasured and therefore invisible" (p. 7). The challenge facing nursing is to create a common language that can be used to organize the phenomena of nursing practice without depersonalizing the patient (Kritek, 1989) and that can be articulated with the standardized languages of medicine and other disciplines. All disciplines must collaborate in the assessment and documentation of health care effectiveness, but all disciplines, including nursing, also must be held accountable for the extent to which their specific interventions achieve desired outcomes.

Currently, neither standardized terminology nor an organizing framework necessary for database development exists for nursing-sensitive patient outcomes (Jennings, 1991). Classification and standardization of nursing-sensitive patient outcomes are necessary if nursing process data are to be included in local, regional, and national databases used to assess provider effectiveness. To achieve this objective, a research team was formed in August 1991 at the University of Iowa to conceptualize, label, and classify nursing-sensitive patient outcomes. The team includes 20 investigators, 4 doctoral students, and 4 consultants. The investigators include nurse researchers, clinical nurse experts, nurse managers, a statistician, and a computer systems specialist.

AIMS OF THE RESEARCH

The aims of Phase I of the research, (a) to identify and resolve conceptual and methodological issues and (b) to develop an initial list of nursing-sensitive patient outcomes and indicators, have been completed. Funding to support Phase I was obtained from Sigma Theta Tau, Gamma Chapter; Sigma Theta Tau International; and the University of Iowa College of Nursing and University of Iowa Hospitals and Clinics Department of Nursing Office of Research. Phase II of the research, funded by the National Institute of Nursing (NINR), aims (a) to place the outcomes and indicators within revised Medical Outcomes Study (MOS) and broad nursing outcome categories; (b) to refine the list of outcomes and indicators through concept analysis (Walker & Avant, 1988; Westra & Rodgers, 1991), assess their validity and nursing sensitivity, and develop definitions; (c) to field-test the initial list of nursing-sensitive outcomes and indicators in four settings; and (d) to organize the list of nursing-sensitive patient outcomes and indicators in a classification structure. It is anticipated that the nursing-sensitive patient outcomes classification, when complete, will contain patient outcomes, indicators, and measures at five or six levels of abstraction (Table 2.2).

CONCEPTUAL ISSUES

Initially, conceptual and methodological issues were identified and resolved so that the work of developing outcome labels and indicators could begin. First, it was important to determine the unit of analysis for the outcomes identified in this study. Although it is recognized that outcomes of interest to nursing include those that characterize individual patients, patient aggregates, organizations, and communities, the current project focuses only on individual patients and families or significant others. This decision recognizes the centrality of individual patient information for the development of databases. Data about groups of patients with a specific medical or nursing diagnosis or in a particular setting, unit, or organization are derived from aggregating data characterizing individual patients.

Second, nursing-sensitive patient outcomes were conceptually defined. Like nursing diagnoses, nursing-sensitive patient outcomes characterize patient states or behaviors, including patient perceptions and subjective states (Erben, Franzkowiak, & Wenzel, 1992), as opposed to the nursing behaviors that are a focus of research in many nursing intervention studies (cf. Iowa Intervention Project, 1992). For this study, a nursing-sensitive patient outcome is defined as

TABLE 2.2 Levels of Outcomes in the Nursing-Sensitive Patient Outcomes
          Classification

Level of Abstraction	Classification
Highest	Nursing-sensitive outcome categories
High-middle	Nursing-sensitive outcome classes
Middle	Nursing-sensitive outcome labels
Low-middle	Nursing-sensitive outcome labels
Lowest	Nursing-sensitive outcome indicators
Empirical	Measurement activities for outcomes

a variable patient or family state, condition, or perception responsive to nursing
intervention and conceptualized at middle levels of abstraction (e.g., mobility
level, nutritional status, health attitudes). Nursing-sensitive outcome indicators are variable patient states, behaviors, or perceptions, conceptualized at a
low level of abstraction, that are responsive to nursing and used for determining a patient outcome (e.g., for mobility level, possible indicators could be joint
movement, transfer performance, ambulation: walking).

Another conceptual issue was how to state outcomes. To facilitate measurement of change, outcomes are conceptualized and stated as nonevaluative,
variable patient states. Thus the standardized outcome labels describe patient states that vary and can be measured and compared to a baseline over
time. As Bond and Thomas (1991) noted, preset outcomes that require change
are not necessary. Unintended consequences of nursing interventions and
maintenance of steady states also are valid and may be desirable outcomes
(Bond & Thomas, 1991). Therefore nursing-sensitive patient outcomes in this
study are *not* stated as goals, although the outcomes and indicators can be used
to set goals for specific patients or populations, with baseline status and
progress assessed over time. These decisions resulted in rules for writing
nursing-sensitive patient outcome labels, outlined in Table 2.3.

To be useful for assessing the effectiveness of nursing, there must be clear
theoretical, research, or practice evidence that the outcomes are responsive to
nursing intervention. This does not mean that all outcomes must be influenced
by nursing alone. Clearly, most outcomes are influenced by the interventions
of several disciplines. However, some outcomes and indicators are more responsive to the interventions of specific disciplines, and it is those most

TABLE 2.3 Rules for Standardization of Nursing-Sensitive Outcomes

An outcome label is stated in nonevaluative terms rather than as a decreased, increased, or improved state.

An outcome label is *not* stated as a nursing diagnosis.

An outcome label does *not* describe a nurse behavior or intervention.

An outcome label describes a patient state that is inherently variable and can be measured and quantified.

An outcome label is conceptualized and stated at a middle level of abstraction. Colons are used to make broader concept labels more specific; however, the broader label is stated first, with the colon and more specific label following (e.g., "nutritional status: intake" or "nutritional status: energy level").

sensitive to nursing interventions that must be identified. Selecting outcomes from nursing literature, research, and clinical systems and having nurse experts rate nursing's influence on outcome achievement is a first step in identifying nursing-sensitive patient outcomes. Further validation of sensitivity will occur as standardized languages are available to allow for the study of linkages among nursing structure, process, and patient outcomes.

Outcomes and indicators are being developed at several levels of abstraction (see Table 2.2) so that they can be used for different purposes (e.g., evaluation of specific nursing interventions with individual patients; comparison of outcomes across populations, settings, and individual providers; applicability to different states of health/illness). Although most of the outcomes and indicators developed in the current project are specific to the resolution of nursing diagnoses or pathology, generic outcomes, such as patient satisfaction with nursing, are also important to classify, as are those that characterize patient aggregates, organizations, and communities (Johnson & Maas, 1994).

Combinations of inductive and deductive and qualitative and quantitative strategies are being used for the development of the classification of nursing-sensitive patient outcomes. In taxonomy development, concept development is intertwined with conceptual framework development, requiring both inductive and deductive approaches (Suppe & Jacox, 1985). Thus integration of quantitative and qualitative methods for identification and testing of nursing-sensitive patient outcomes is needed (Erben et al., 1992). The qualitative and classification methods used for the research are modeled after, but not entirely the same as, those of the Nursing Interventions Classification (NIC) project (Cohen et al., 1991; Iowa Intervention Project, 1992).

DEVELOPMENT OF OUTCOME LABELS

The second step was to develop an initial list of patient outcomes currently used in nursing. A sampling plan, representative of clinical emphases, settings, and patient age groups, was developed to ensure representativeness and comprehensiveness of the outcome statements. Sources were selected to represent medical/surgical, critical care, maternal/child, rehabilitation, and mental health clinical practice; acute care, nursing home, community, and ambulatory settings; and elderly, adult, child, and infant populations. The following criteria were used to select sources: (a) presents clear statements describing specific states or behaviors of patients/families, (b) includes a comprehensive list of outcome statements, (c) presents measurable outcome statements, and (d) describes outcome statements specifically designed to evaluate nursing interventions.

More than 4,500 outcome statements were extracted from 18 sources to develop an initial list of 282 nursing-sensitive patient outcomes and indicators. These outcome statements were at varied levels of abstraction and were usually stated as goals or standards (e.g., from broad statements such as prevention of complications or maintenance of optimal activity level, to midlevel statements such as knowledge of proper dressing care, to very specific statements such as "cardiac index 2.5 to 4.0 liters/minute." One hundred and fifty to 250 of these outcome statements were distributed to each member of the research team in exercises. Each team member clustered similar statements and developed an outcome label for the concept reflected in the cluster. Twenty exercises were determined sufficient because outcome statements for areas identified in the sampling scheme were saturated. The labels and associated outcome statements from each exercise and team member were entered into a computer database using Paradox. As the list of labels and outcome statements grew, the labels were reviewed to eliminate redundancy and to standardize semantics and grammar according to the rules in Table 2.3. Table 2.4 contains examples of the outcome labels and associated outcome statements on the initial list.

From 3 to 25 outcome statements were grouped under each of the outcome labels and used as the basis for development of indicators for each of the outcome labels. To refine the labels and outcome statements and to identify nursing-sensitive outcomes and indicators not included, the outcome labels were placed within the following eight broad categories based on the Medical Outcomes Study (MOS) (Tarlov et al., 1989) and outcome categories identified in nursing literature (Lang & Clinton, 1984; Marek, 1989): physiological status, psychological/cognitive status, social and role status, physical functional status, safety status, family caregiver status, health attitudes/knowledge/behavior, and perceived well-being. A revised Delphi process with members of the research

TABLE 2.4 Examples of Outcomes and Associated Outcome Statements on Initial
List Prior to Content Analysis and Validation

Label	Outcome Statement
Mobility level: ambulation	Progressive moderate exercising and ambulation Increased ambulation daily
Nutritional status	Decreased appetite improved Patient consumes most of food on meal tray
Pain level	Verbalizes relief and/or absence of pain Absence of associated pain

team was used to assign each outcome label to one of the eight categories. Each of the broad categories was then assigned to one of eight focus groups for concept analysis, development and refinement of outcome labels and indicators, and initial validation of nursing sensitivity.

CONCEPT ANALYSIS

Focus groups have two to four research team members each and are chaired by doctorally prepared investigators. Expert clinicians were added to each group to assist with the work. To refine labels and indicators, the focus groups reviewed nursing and allied research, instruments measuring the outcome concepts, and other pertinent work. Each focus group (a) reviewed the outcome labels in their category, collapsed similar labels as appropriate, and added new labels as needed, with 7 new outcome labels added and approximately 100 labels collapsed; (b) standardized the language of the outcome label and developed a definition for the label based on the concept analysis; (c) refined each outcome statement in the initial list and developed additional outcome statements based on the literature review and concept analysis; (d) presented a summary of the concept analysis, the outcome label, the definition, and indicators to the research team for review and adoption for field testing; (e) provided information about the frequency of use of each outcome label in nursing; and (f) developed a list of references for each label. Examples of refined nursing-sensitive outcomes and indicators are shown in Table 2.5 with examples of rudimentary measurement scales.

A survey of master's-prepared clinical nurse experts, representing a cross section of clinical emphases, settings, and client age groups, is being done to validate the content of the patient outcomes and indicators and to estimate their sensitivity to nursing interventions. A revision of Fehring's (1986, 1987)

TABLE 2.5 Selected Examples of Refined Nursing-Sensitive Outcomes and Indicators

Outcome and Definition	Indicators	Scale		
Ambulation:		Not Adequate		Adequate
Walking Performance	Gait effectiveness			
The ability to walk	Walking speed			
from place to place	Walking distance			
	Weight bearing			
		Never	Sometimes	Always
	Assistive devices required			
	Human assistance needed			
Nutritional Status		Below Requirements	Meets Requirements	Exceeds Requirements
The proportion of	Nutrient intake			
nutrients available	Food and fluid intake			
to meet metabolic	Energy level			
needs	Body mass: weight			
	Serum albumin			
	Lymphocyte count			
	Hemoglobin			
	Hematocrit			
	Urinary urea nitrogen			
Nutritional Status:		Below Requirements	Meets Requirements	Exceeds Requirements
Food and Fluid Intake	Oral food intake			
The amount of food and	Tube feeding intake			
fluid taken into the body	Oral fluid intake			
over a 20-hour period	Parenteral fluid intake			
Pain Level				Worst Possible
Reported and/or exhibited	Verbal expression of	None		
state of physical discomfort	pain intensity			
	Verbal expression of percentage of body affected	0%		100%
	Verbal expression of frequency of pain	Rare		Constant
	Verbal expression of length of pain episodes	Brief		Continuous
	Vocalizations (e.g., crying, moaning, whimpering)	None		Continuous
	Facial expressions (e.g., grimacing, clenched teeth)			
	Protective body posture/ positions			
	Restless movements			
	Muscle tension			
		Greatly Increased		Greatly Decreased
	Respiratory rate			
	Heart rate			
	Blood pressure			
	Pupil size			
	Perspiration			
	Appetite			
	Medication use			

SOURCE: Nursing-Sensitive Outcomes Classification (NOC), University of Iowa College of Nursing.

methodology for assessing content validity of nursing diagnoses has been piloted to estimate both content validity and sensitivity to nursing interventions. Concept analysis is nearing completion, and a refined list of nursing-sensitive patient outcomes will soon be published and available for field testing.

CONTINUED WORK

Following completion of the validation surveys, the list of nursing-sensitive patient outcomes and indicators will be field tested in four sites: (a) a tertiary, acute care hospital; (b) an intermediate acute care hospital; (c) a nursing home; and (d) a home care nursing agency. Throughout the field testing, the following will be assessed: (a) compatibility of the outcomes and indicators with clinical information systems; (b) use of the outcomes and indicators by practicing clinical nurses; (c) use of the outcomes and indicators for nursing administrative and management quality assessment purposes; (d) linkages among nurses' documentation of diagnoses, interventions, and outcomes; and (e) pilot results of alternative measurement procedures.

Finally, similarity-dissimilarity analysis, using hierarchical clustering procedures, will be conducted to develop the nursing-sensitive outcomes classification structure. The classification structure will (a) relate outcomes and indicators in terms of levels of abstraction and (b) group outcomes and indicators according to some rules that define commonalities within the groups. As stated, the classification is expected to have five or six increasingly specific levels of outcomes (Table 2.2).

IMPLICATIONS FOR NURSE
ADMINISTRATORS AND MANAGERS

The Nursing-Sensitive Outcomes Classification (NOC) will be the first comprehensive list of standardized outcome labels, definitions, and indicators to describe patient outcomes influenced by nursing care. It will provide standardized outcomes to complete the nursing process elements of the Nursing Minimum Data Set (NMDS). Although the NMDS was developed in the 1980s, relatively little progress has been made toward consistent inclusion of these elements in clinical and management nursing information systems (Simpson, 1993). Lack of standardized languages for the nursing process elements of the NMDS has been a major reason for slow progress. It is hoped that the current NOC work, as well as standardization of nursing diagnoses (NANDA) and nursing interventions (NIC), will stimulate greater use of the NMDS. Consistent use of the NMDS will provide nurse managers with information useful for evaluating the impact of nursing on the attainment of organizational goals. It will also provide data that nurses can use to influence policy formulation.

This research will provide the common language essential for the evaluation of clinical and management interventions in nursing. The use of a common language in clinical practice settings will provide a rich database for comparison of patient outcomes across clinical settings and sites and within or across populations of patients grouped by medical diagnoses, nursing diagnoses, other patient characteristics, or organizational characteristics. It will provide data necessary for analyzing the relationships between nursing interventions and patient outcomes with large patient populations in multisite studies. This information is essential for nursing to describe its effectiveness and value to other health care workers, administrators, policy makers, and consumers.

Development of outcomes as neutral concepts that can be measured on a continuum rather than as expected standards will facilitate the identification and analysis of outcomes currently being achieved for specific populations. It will also facilitate the identification of patient or organizational characteristics that influence outcome attainment. Assessment of the level of outcomes over time provides much more useful information than just documenting whether outcomes are achieved. For example, patients can be aggregated by a nursing diagnosis, and differences in level of outcome achievement can be analyzed by personal characteristics such as age, gender, or functional status or by organizational characteristics such as staff mix, unit size, or ratio of registered nurses to patients. This information can assist nurse managers and clinicians in developing realistic standards for specific patient populations. Standards can be consistent with the currently achieved outcomes if the outcome level is satisfactory, or they can reflect desired, higher levels of achievement, in which case the nurse manager will have an understanding of the amount of improvement needed to attain such outcomes. This will be quite different from the usual practice of setting standards without adequate knowledge of whether the standard is actually achieved or is too low or too high. Development of outcomes as variables also encourages the identification of specific goals for each patient. The nurse can specify the desired level of achievement for each patient based upon the initial assessment and then measure the actual level of achievement. Another important application of measuring outcomes as variables is that they are more useful for evaluating the effects of nursing care over time than at a single point in time: In other words, one can trace and graph the patient's status over a prolonged period within and across care settings.

NOC will be available for inclusion in nursing clinical data sets in all settings and in large regional and national data sets. Data from individual patients and various settings can be aggregated to determine the levels at which outcomes are most commonly achieved for patients with a specific medical or nursing diagnosis. Accumulation of this more detailed information about the effectiveness or lack of effectiveness of nursing interventions will add to nursing knowledge and will allow nursing to identify areas of practice that need improvement.

In summary, once nurse administrators have included the outcomes and indicators in clinical data sets, they will have multiple uses. They can be used to set expected outcome goals for nursing interventions, evaluate nursing interventions for individual patients/clients, and assist in clinical decision making. Nurse administrators and managers can use them to evaluate nursing management and clinical interventions for aggregates of patients/clients and to describe patterns of patient outcomes across settings, patient aggregates, and regions of the United States. This allows nursing effectiveness to be longitudinally monitored on the basis of change rather than at a single point in time. Use of the standardized outcomes and indicators will make nursing a more visible and accountable provider in interdisciplinary health care and provide data for nurse administrators' decision making and influence on health policy.

REFERENCES

Agency for Health Care Policy and Research. (1990, September). *AHCPR: Purpose and programs.* Washington, DC: Government Printing Office.

Agency for Health Care Policy and Research. (1991). *Report to Congress: The feasibility of linking research-related data bases to federal and non-federal medical administrative data bases* (AHCPR Pub. No. 91-0003). Rockville, MD: Author.

American Nurses Association. (1977). *Guidelines for review of nursing care at the local level.* Kansas City, KS: Author.

Aydelotte, M. (1962). The use of patient welfare as a criterion measure. *Nursing Research, 11,* 10-14.

Bergman, R. (1993, December 5). The measuring stick. *Hospitals and Health Networks,* pp. 36-38, 40, 42.

Bond, S., & Thomas, L. H. (1991). Issues in measuring outcomes on nursing. *Journal of Advanced Nursing, 16,* 1492-1502.

Brook, H. L. (1989). Practice guidelines and practicing medicine: Are they compatible? *Journal of the American Medical Association, 262,* 3027-3030.

Cohen, M. Z., Kruckeberg, T., McCloskey, J., Bulechek, G., Craft, M. J., Denehy, J., Glick, O., Maas, M., Prophet, C., Tripp-Reimer, T., Carlson, D., & Wyman, M. (1991). Inductive methodology and a research team. *Nursing Outlook, 39*(4), 162-165.

Darby, M. (1993). Kaiser's "Report Care" illustrates promises and pitfalls of a trend. *Report on Medical Guidelines and Outcomes Research, 4*(21), 1, 2, 5.

DeFriese, G. H. (1990). Measuring the effectiveness of medical interventions: New expectations of health services research. *Health Services Research, 25,* 697-708.

Donabedian, A. (1966). Evaluating the quality of medical care. *Milbank Memorial Fund Quarterly, 44*(3), 166-206.

Erben, R., Franzkowiak, P., & Wenzel, E. (1992). Assessment of the outcomes of health intervention. *Social Science and Medicine, 35,* 359-365.

Fehring, R. J. (1986). Validating diagnostic labels: Standardized methodology. In M. E. Hurley (Ed.), *Classification of nursing diagnoses: Proceedings of the sixth conference* (pp. 183-190). St. Louis: C. V. Mosby.

Fehring, R. J. (1987). Methods to validate nursing diagnoses. *Heart and Lung, 16,* 625-629.

Horn, B. J., & Swain, M. A. (1978). *Criterion measures of nursing care* (DHEW Pub. No. PHS 78-3187). Hyattsville, MD: National Center for Health Services Research.

Hover, J., & Zimmer, M. (1978). Nursing quality assurance: The Wisconsin system. *Nursing Outlook, 26,* 242-248.

Iowa Intervention Project. (1992). *Nursing interventions classification (NIC).* St. Louis: C. V. Mosby.

Jennings, B. M. (1991). Patient outcomes research: Seizing the opportunity. *Advances in Nursing Science, 14*(2), 59-72.

Johnson, M., & Maas, M. (1994). Nursing focused patient outcomes: Challenge for the nineties. In J. McCloskey & H. K. Grace (Eds.), *Current issues in nursing* (4th ed., pp. 136-142). St. Louis: C. V. Mosby.

Kritek, P. V. (1989). An introduction to the science and art of taxonomy. In American Nurses Association (Ed.), *Classification systems for describing nursing practice: Working papers* (pp. 6-12). Kansas City, KS: American Nurses Association.

Lang, N. M., & Clinton, J. F. (1984). Assessment of quality of nursing care. *Annual Review of Nursing Research, 2,* 135-163.

Lang, N. M., & Marek, K. D. (1990). The classification of patient outcomes. *Journal of Professional Nursing, 6,* 153-163.

Lange, L. L., & Jacox, A. (1993). Using large data bases in nursing and health policy research. *Journal of Professional Nursing, 9*(4), 204-211.

Lembke, P. A. (1959). A scientific method for medical auditing. Part one. *Hospitals, 33,* 65-71.

Lohr, K. N. (1988). Outcome measurement: Concepts and questions. *Inquiry, 25*(1), 37-50.

Lower, M. S., & Burton, S. (1989). Measuring the impact of nursing interventions on patient outcomes: The challenge of the 1990s. *Journal of Nursing Quality Assurance, 4*(1), 27-34.

Mallison, M. B. (1990). Editorial: Access to invisible expressways. *American Journal of Nursing, 90*(9), 7.

Marek, K. D. (1989). Outcome measurement in nursing. *Journal of Nursing Quality Assurance, 4*(1), 1-9.

Martin, K. S., & Scheet, N. J. (1992). *The Omaha system: Applications for community health nursing.* Philadelphia: W. B. Saunders.

McCloskey, J. C., & Bulechek, G. M. (1994). Standardizing the language for nursing: An overview of the issues. *Nursing Outlook, 42*(2), 56-63.

North American Nursing Diagnosis Association. (1992). *NANDA nursing diagnoses: Definitions and classification 1992-1993.* Philadelphia: Author.

O'Leary, D. (1987). The Joint Commission looks to the future [Editorial]. *Journal of the American Medical Association, 258,* 951-952.

Ozbolt, J. G. (1991, September). *Strategies for building nursing databases for effectiveness research.* Abstract of paper presented at conference, Patient Outcomes Research: Examining the Effectiveness of Nursing Practice, Rockville, MD.

Roper, W. L. (1990). Seeking effectiveness in health care: The federal perspective. *Internist, 31*(1), 9-10.

Roper, W. L., Winkenwerder, W., Hackbarth, G. M., & Krakauer, H. (1988). Effectiveness in health care and initiative to evaluate and improve medical practice. *New England Journal of Medicine, 319,* 1197-1202.

Saba, B. K., O'Hare, A., Zuckerman, A. E., Boondasj, J., Levine, E., & Oatway, D. M. (1991). A nursing intervention taxonomy for home health care. *Nursing and Healthcare, 12*(6), 296-299.

Salive, M. E., Mayfield, J. A., & Weissman, N. W. (1990). Patient outcomes research teams and the Agency for Health Care Policy and Research. *Health Services Research, 25,* 697-708.

Simpson, R. L. (1993). A nursing management minimum data set. *Nursing Management, 24*(4), 24-25.

Skolnick, A. A. (1993). Joint Commission will collect, publicize outcomes. *Journal of the American Medical Association, 270,* 165-171.

Suppe, F., & Jacox, A. K. (1985). Philosophy of science and the development of nursing theory. *Annual Review of Nursing Research, 3,* 241-267.

Tarlov, A. R., Ware, J. E., Greenfield, S., Nelson, E. C., Perrin, E., & Zubkoff, M. (1989). The Medical Outcomes Study: An application of methods for monitoring the results of medical care. *Journal of the American Medical Association, 262,* 925-930.

Walker, A. O., & Avant, K. C. (1988). *Strategies for theory construction in nursing* (2nd ed.). Norwalk, CT: Appleton & Lange.

Wennberg, J., & Giltelsohn, A. (1973). Small area variations in health care delivery. *Science, 182,* 1102-1108.

Werley, H. H., & Lang, N. M. (Eds.). (1988). *Identification of the Nursing Minimum Data Set.* New York: Springer.

Westra, B. L., & Rodgers, B. L. (1991). The concept of integration: A foundation for evaluating outcomes of nursing care. *Journal of Professional Nursing, 7,* 277-282.

CHAPTER 3

Nurse Roles in Primary Care: Providing Leadership for Health Care Reform

Reni Courtney

Nurse administrators will face many challenges in a reformed health care system. One of these challenges will involve the transition of a hospital-focused health care system to a system that emphasizes community-based primary care. This chapter provides an overview of primary care and primary care models and describes the roles of nurses in basic and advanced practice in primary care settings. Special emphasis is placed on the nurse administrator role and the knowledge and skills required for administration of primary health care that is grounded in a professional nursing model.

A DAY IN THE LIFE OF . . .

Nurse Ramirez, RN, works in the health care program of a Hispanic-neighborhood-based Community Partnership Center (CPC) that is one of 10 such centers administered by an urban health plan. Nurse Ramirez is leaving Mrs. Sanchez's home following a home visit. She is pleased with the Sanchez family's progress. Nurse Ramirez has been working with the Sanchez family for several months after meeting Mrs. Sanchez at the Parent Health Advocates group that Nurse Ramirez facilitates on a weekly basis at the local middle school. At the first meeting, Nurse Ramirez was concerned about Mrs. Sanchez when she mentioned how difficult things had been since her husband left and how hard it was for the family to pay rent and buy groceries. Nurse Ramirez asked her if she would like to visit with a community worker who lived in the neighborhood and who might be able to help her with some problems. The community worker visited weekly for 1 month and helped the family to learn about emergency assistance and other resources. Nurse Ramirez also invited Mrs. Sanchez to bring her family to the CPC to participate in the Family Assessment Program managed by Nurse Ramirez and the family nurse practitioner (FNP). All family members received screening exams to determine problems, risks, and strengths. At the CPC, Mrs. Sanchez continues to receive well-woman care from the FNP and weekly counseling from the nurse therapist. Her children are also seen by the FNP as their primary care provider who coordinates services with the RN and the three community workers who are on her team.

After 3 months in the Parent Health Advocates group, the parents wanted to begin a teen group for their children. Nurse Ramirez worked with the parents and two teens to plan this group. She also trained the teen leaders to facilitate small groups. The teen group has been very successful and averages 10 teens who have been meeting weekly for 2 months.

Nurse Ramirez's next appointment is with four school nurses, who are employed by the CPC, to plan how to coordinate resources and programs for the next semester. The last appointment of the day is the monthly meeting of the community board that oversees all operations of the CPC and works actively to organize neighborhood residents into special-interest action groups. One of the citizen action groups that Nurse Ramirez works with is developing a neighborhood survey to determine which residents would be interested in literacy classes and health education programs. She looks forward to seeing the FNP, the community workers, and the nurse administrator at the meeting. She knows she will be able to visit also with the director of the housing program, local police officers, school principals, and other community leaders at the meeting.

INTRODUCTION

The U.S. health care system operates on the basis of a biomedical model that is disease focused, oriented to individuals, and reductionistic (Allan & Hall, 1988). Although the United States spends 14% of its GNP on health care services, it does not achieve the same level of health as other industrialized countries that spend only half as much. Even a cautious analyst would conclude that the U.S. health care system is in need of reform.

Winston Churchill has said, "You can always count on Americans to do the right thing—after they have tried everything else." Doing the right thing requires that we recognize that the health care system, including health professions education, financing mechanisms, health care priorities, and delivery systems, must be revised to address existing and emerging societal needs. For years we have known in the United States that there are many important determinants of health, such as socioeconomic, cultural, and psychological factors. Yet we have continued to support a health care system that focuses almost exclusively on the delivery of biomedical services to individuals, ignoring all we know about the factors that influence health in populations (Allan & Hall, 1988). While the rest of the world increasingly focuses on the development and delivery of multifaceted primary care health services that are population based, the United States continues to deliver mostly high-tech medical services to the individual. The medical model and its derived medical services have an important place in the health care system but are inadequate to prevent disease, address a full range of health problems, or promote health.

The United States requires new thinking to build a more sensible, cost-effective, equitable health care system. The American Nurses Association (ANA; 1991b) has proposed such a system in its Agenda for Health Care Reform, in which it has called for a restructured health care system that

> Enhances consumer access to services by delivering primary health care in community-based settings.
> Fosters consumer responsibility for personal health, self care, and informed decision-making in selecting health care services.
> Facilitates utilization of the most cost-effective providers and therapeutic options in the most appropriate settings. (p. 2)

ANA's plan for a reformed system requires the transformation of the present illness system to one that emphasizes primary care, which will serve as the broad foundation for all other services.

The Community Partnership Center (CPC) described in the opening scenario is based on a broad conception of health such as that advocated by the ANA. The CPC recognizes the influence of physical, mental, social, and political health determinants in addition to biomedical. Although many different professionals are required to form partnerships with community members to create and implement the type of organization represented by the CPC, professional nurses are the ideal professionals to form the core. Nurse administrators of vision and courage are needed to create and to assume leadership roles in these types of organizations. This chapter provides an overview of primary care and primary care models and describes the roles of nurses in basic and advanced practice in primary care settings. Special emphasis is placed on the nurse administrator role and the knowledge and skills required for administration of primary health care delivery that is grounded in a professional nursing model.

OVERVIEW OF PRIMARY CARE

Primary care has received dramatic attention in recent discussions of health care reform and is expected to provide a major foundation to a reformed health care system (ANA, 1991b; Eckholm, 1993; Starr, 1992). What exactly is primary care, and is there a common understanding of this area of practice?

Primary Care Definitions

The theoretical foundations of primary care are not well developed, and a variety of concepts and definitions abound. *Primary care* has been defined in the literature in many ways, including a type of care, a level of service, a set of characteristics, a group of specialties or disciplines, a list of services, and a location for service (Agency for Health Care Policy and Research [AHCPR], 1993).

A well-known definition of *primary care* described it as

> a person's first contact in any given episode of illness with the health care system that leads to a decision of what must be done to help resolve this problem; and . . . the responsibility for the continuum of care, i.e., maintenance of health, evaluation and management of symptoms and appropriate referrals. (U.S. Dept. of Health, Education, and Welfare, 1971, p. 8)

A similar description of primary care was proposed in one of the earliest reports on primary care (Millis, 1966). Starfield (1992) defined *primary care* as "the assumption of longitudinal responsibility for the patient, regardless of the presence or absence of disease; and the integration of physical, psychological, and social aspects of health to the limits of the health personnel's capabilities" (p. 9). An ANA Fact Sheet (1991a) defined *primary care* as "a holistic approach to health care initiated at the client's first entry into the health care system. . . . Continuous and comprehensive, primary health care entails coordination of all the services necessary for health promotion, maintenance, rehabilitation, and the prevention of disease and disability" (p. 1).

There are many other definitions of *primary care,* but all are similar in that they emphasize first-contact care, responsibility for longitudinal care, and a focus on person-centered care. The identification of the major characteristics of primary care were first presented in an Institute of Medicine (IOM) report: first contact, comprehensiveness, continuity, coordination, accessibility, and accountability (IOM, 1978). It is these characteristics, particularly those of continuous, comprehensive, and coordinated care, that differentiate primary care from the episodic care that is delivered in other ambulatory settings such as the emergency department or minor treatment centers.

The IOM Committee on the Future of Primary Care (IOM, 1994) has proposed the following provisional definition of *primary care:* "Primary care is the provision of integrated, accessible health care services by clinicians who are accountable for addressing a large majority of personal health care needs, developing a sustained partnership with patients, and practicing in the context of family and community" (p. 1).

The committee will continue its 2-year study of primary care to determine a final definition and key recommendations for primary care.

Primary Care Models

Several conceptualizations and/or models of primary care exist. Selected models, including primary health care (PHC), primary medical care (PMC), community-oriented primary care (COPC), and community partnership primary care (CPPC), are discussed briefly here.

PHC and PMC

It is essential to differentiate the concepts of primary health care (PHC) and primary medical care (PMC), as can be seen in Figure 3.1. PHC is a much broader concept of primary care than PMC and encompasses services, support, and facilitation by health professionals to promote the health and foster the empowerment of individuals, families, and the community (Courtney, 1995). In 1978, the World Health Organization published a definition of *PHC* as follows:

> Essential health care based on practical, scientifically sound, and socially acceptable methods and technology made universally accessible to individuals and families in the community by means acceptable to them and at a cost that the community and country can afford to maintain at every stage of their development in a spirit of self-reliance and self-determination. It forms an integral part of both the country's health system of which it is the central function and the main focus of the overall social and economic development of the community. It is the first level of contact of individuals, the family and the community with the national health system, bringing health care as close as possible where people live and work and constitutes the first element of a continuing health care process. (p. 3)

This definition of *PHC* contrasts markedly with that of *PMC,* which is generally understood to be the delivery of first-contact medicine, largely through office-based care (Frenk, Gonzalez-Block, & Alvarez-Manilla, 1990; Starfield, 1992).

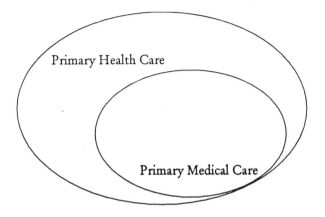

Figure 3.1. Comparison of Primary Health Care With Primary Medical Care

Policy makers typically mean PMC when they use the term *primary care,* although it is unlikely that they are aware of distinctions regarding the nature of primary care. Policy makers must be educated to understand that PMC is only a component of broader health strategies and interventions known as PHC. They must also learn that careful analysis of the public's health has revealed that the contribution of medical care to health is very small in modern nations (Fuchs, 1986). Health policy that will result in a healthier public must include areas for action that are outside the traditional realm of medical care (Meyer & Silow-Carroll, 1993).

Medicine has long been recognized as providing leadership in the area of primary care. However, increasingly nurses and the community, drawing on a professional nursing model, have begun to develop a PHC system that truly focuses on health, not just disease.

COPC

A model of primary care that has received attention in the past decade is entitled *community-oriented primary care,* or COPC (IOM, 1984). COPC is primary care that extends beyond an individual focus to include principles of public health, specifically integrating the science of epidemiology into primary care. There are two major differences between primary care and COPC: In COPC, (a) the target population must be defined, and (b) activities must be developed that systematically address the health problems of that population as defined through epidemiology (Nutting, 1987).

COPC is the first primary care model to recommend inclusion of public health science and a focus on the health of aggregates. This is important to note because many policy makers and professionals incorrectly use the terms *primary care, community health,* and *community-based care* synonymously. Usually, primary care and/or care delivered in community-based settings is not population based, meaning that a public health focus on the group or aggregates served is not a typical component. Rather, services are provided ad hoc to individuals who present themselves for care. Because COPC focuses on population-based care, it will be increasingly emphasized as a important model in a health care system focused on managed care with a primary care emphasis.

CPPC

The author has been involved in developing and testing a model of primary care that builds on principles of COPC yet extends beyond this model (Courtney, 1995). In CPPC, primary care is integrated not only with a population-based focus, as is COPC, but also with a new area for practice, community development. *Community development* is defined broadly as a process in which the community organizes itself to identify and solve its own problems. In CPPC, health professionals do not focus only on the health care delivery system and/or services; they develop partnerships in which they participate with and facilitate community members to define, explore, and prioritize issues of concern. Community members are supported to determine their desired roles, responsibilities, and strategies to empower their community and to promote its health and well-being. Community members may invite health professionals to participate in these efforts as partners. In this way, health professionals begin to be involved in primary prevention strategies developed and driven by community members. Together, community members and health professionals focus on strengthening the community, which is the root of health, rather than emphasizing only the health care system. CPPC's emphasis on fostering empowerment of individuals, groups, and the community is expected to result ultimately in improved health and stronger communities. The CPPC model recognizes that promoting a healthier community requires more than providing clinical services; actions by community members and health professionals must be directed toward other important determinants of health.

Nursing has both the opportunity and the challenge to participate in designing new systems of care that move beyond existing models of primary care. These new systems of care must move beyond a medical paradigm to include partnerships with communities and grassroots citizens' groups, an emphasis on health promotion and disease prevention that will result in more empowered citizens with increased self-responsibility for health, and increased collaboration among existing health and human services. The new paradigm must be based on a broad conception of health, such as that promulgated over the years by professional nursing.

Primary Care Providers

Many nurses provide primary care services. The focus of advanced-practice nurses (APNs) such as nurse practitioners (NPs) and certified nurse midwives (CNMs) is primary care, with approximately 50,000 NPs and 7,500 CNMs currently prepared (Health Resources and Services Administration [HRSA], 1994). A small percentage of the 58,000 clinical nurse specialists (CNSs) is also educated in the specialty of primary care. Approximately 400,000 registered nurses, 23% of the RN workforce, provide primary care services in schools, public health clinics, occupational health settings, and other community-based, ambulatory settings (HRSA, 1994). This cadre of nurse primary care providers could be very quickly supplemented from the current ranks of CNSs and RNs after they receive additional education in primary care and community health.

Scrutiny of the physician workforce has been intense as plans for health care reform are developed. Of the approximately 600,000 physicians in the United States, over two thirds are now specialists, leaving only 27% or approximately 200,000 physicians in primary care disciplines such as family practice, pediatrics, and general medicine (Council on Graduate Medical Education, Petersdorf, 1992). Currently, only 14% of medical school graduates choose primary care fields, despite the large amounts of federal funds that have been targeted to family practice and other primary care specialties over the past two decades (Colwill, 1992). A review of the American Medical Association registry of physicians in practice revealed the surprising finding that the discipline of family medicine had not grown at all during the past 25 years despite extensive effort to promote this area of practice (Petersdorf, 1993).

The Council on Graduate Medical Education (COGME; 1992) issued a recent report calling for primary care physicians to constitute 50% of the physician workforce. However, the council predicted that it will take until the year 2040 before this percentage of primary care physicians can be achieved.

Many nurse leaders and even medical leaders question the assumptions that underlie the COGME recommendation. Focusing only on the primary care physician workforce ignores other providers such as APNs, RNs, and physician assistants, who provide a significant portion of primary care services. If the health care system is significantly restructured to include emphasis on primary care, then large numbers of primary care providers will be needed immediately, not 45 years from now. The ideal primary care provider will be one who possesses a broad range of skills to provide health promotion and disease prevention care in addition to illness care. The nurse practitioner is this ideal provider, joined by CNMs, other APNs, and RNs.

For example, it is critical for policy makers to know that nurse practitioners can be prepared at approximately one sixth the cost of preparing a primary care physician and in approximately one half the time. In addition, nurse practitioners have been determined through countless studies to provide anywhere from 65% to 90% of primary care without need for physician consultation (Office of Technology Assessment [OTA], 1986). NP scope of practice is remarkably similar to that of primary care physicians when the medical dimension of practice is considered (Safriet, 1992). Finally, their care has received close scrutiny over a 25-year period, and policy makers have concluded that NPs and CNMs, "within their areas of competence, provide care whose quality is equivalent to that care provided by physicians" (OTA, 1986, p. 5). Further, "NPs and CNMs are more adept than physicians at providing services that depend on communication with patients and preventive actions" (OTA, 1986, p. 6).

Nurse leaders must continue to proclaim loudly that nurses and nurse practitioners are the most significant part of the formula for increasing quality primary care health services in the United States. Fortunately, legislators and a growing number of policy makers do recognize and promote the nurse's role in health care reform.

Nurses, nurse practitioners, and other APNs must join with other colleagues and the community to meet the challenges ahead in a reformed system. Nurses, however, bring formidable contributions to the health care system and must be bold and persistent in providing leadership to the formulation of a new system.

NURSE ROLES IN PRIMARY CARE

There are a variety of roles for nurses in primary care. The roles of RNs, APNs, and nurse administrators are discussed here. Although many of these nurses have functioned in primary care for years, health care reform will force a renewed consideration of practice roles and responsibilities using the key criteria of access, quality, and costs. Nursing cannot assume that current roles will continue as they have in the past. Therefore this section raises questions and issues regarding the roles of each group. The nursing profession must work diligently and creatively to address these issues.

RNs in Primary Care

RNs have long been recognized for the essential roles they assume in the health care system. They are known for their comprehensive approach to patient care that involves highly developed clinical skills, an emphasis on patient education and counseling, and a focus on promoting health and preventing disease. RNs' special skills in the area of coordination of care and case management are well known. These skills will be directly applicable to primary care practice. However, RNs must develop additional knowledge and skills for effective practice in a new arena.

It is well documented that over 66% of all RNs practice in hospitals (HRSA, 1994). With health care reform, as hospitals downsize and community-based settings proliferate, RNs will move increasingly to the community setting. Nursing practice that focuses on families, groups, and the community, with an emphasis on prevention and wellness, contrasts sharply with the individual, illness focus of many nurses in the acute care setting.

Many RNs who move into primary care and community health practices must learn skills not only for typical primary care but develop a new skill set to enable them to implement new, creative approaches to health promotion and community-based care. Examples of required knowledge and skills in typical primary care that experienced acute care nurses may need to strengthen include those listed in Table 3.1. Examples of new knowledge and skills that RNs do not typically possess but that will be required for practice in newer models of primary care such as COPC and CPPC that incorporate community health and community development are shown in Table 3.2.

Current roles of the RN in primary care and in community health may or may not align well with a reformed health care system. What should be the role(s) of RNs in community-based settings? Should they manage panels of individuals and families in collaboration with APNs and physicians? Should they have significant responsibilities for community practice, as demonstrated in the opening scenario, or should they be more involved in the delivery of traditional clinical services? Should they supervise a team of community workers, indigenous workers who provide outreach and support services in the neighborhood, or would this be better managed by social workers?

How will RN roles compare with the roles of other health professionals? Will RNs be more involved in health education and health promotion programs, or will health educators become more prominent? How will RN roles compare with social worker roles in primary care settings? What are unique responsibilities that will require the clinical skills and/or comprehensive focus of an RN? What responsibilities and/or tasks can be delegated to LVNs or other health

TABLE 3.1 Selected Examples of Required RN Knowledge for Primary Care

- Health care problems not commonly seen in acute care settings, such as otitis media and skin rashes
- Undifferentiated problems presented at initial visits that have not yet been diagnosed
- Conducting of comprehensive health assessments for all ages
- Medications used in primary care
- Provision of health education and health promotion counseling
- Community resources and community networks
- Extension of clinical care into the community to include home visits, screening, and case finding
- Case management to include community referrals and coordination of multiple sources of care
- Understanding of epidemiologic data about the community and various subgroups
- Participation in developing community diagnosis
- Targeted outreach to high-risk groups
- Community health education involving groups
- Screening programs and case finding

professionals? What will be the costs for RN practice in community-based settings?

What will be the differences between the roles of associate-degree and baccalaureate-degree nurses in primary care settings? It is important to emphasize that baccalaureate-prepared nurses (BSNs) have received significant

TABLE 3.2 New Knowledge in Community Development for RNs

- Understanding of a community development process
- Knowledge of techniques to develop partnerships between health professionals and community members
- Skill in networking with community agencies, groups, and leaders to develop collaborative relationships
- Design of community health promotion projects
- Identification and mobilization of natural helpers in the community
- Conducting of focus groups
- Small-group formation and facilitation
- Program development and evaluation
- Community development and community empowerment approaches developed in partnership with community members

instruction in community health practice, in contrast to associate-degree nurses (ADNs). What will be the roles for each type of nurse, particularly when one considers that more ADNs than BSNs may be displaced from the hospital? How will administrators determine RN roles in the short term before longer term evaluation data are available regarding these roles in community-based settings?

The relationship between the scope of practice for APNs and that for baccalaureate nurses will receive increased scrutiny in primary care. Already there are NPs who assert that RNs do not provide primary care because these NPs define *primary care* in a way that requires APNs. Public health nurses and school nurses claim that they have always practiced primary care. This dispute raises the larger question of what we really mean by *primary care*. What aspects of primary care require advanced practitioners, and what areas can be addressed by RNs? It is important to achieve role clarity regarding the unique roles for APNs and RNs in primary care and to determine to what extent shared roles are acceptable and/or cost-effective. What role expansion for RNs could or should occur before the point of advanced practice and the requirement for graduate education?

As nursing moves increasingly into the field of primary care, how will RN education be altered at the baccalaureate- and associate-degree levels? Will nursing maintain both the BSN and ADN levels? As APNs increasingly demonstrate their broad scope of practice in primary care settings, will there be an insatiable demand for nurses at this level rather than the BSN? Will nursing decide that the generic professional degree should be the master's rather than the bachelor's?

Administrators will be concerned with roles other than nursing roles. How can nonprofessional, nonlicensed staff such as community workers be best used in primary care systems? What are the roles for volunteers and community members in community-based settings? How can they provide leadership or be involved in neighborhood systems of care? Who will determine the community's role?

Nurse administrators, educators, and practitioners must join with the community to determine acceptable and creative answers to the above questions. Researchers must design the critical studies that will provide essential data about RN and other roles in community-based settings. Most important, nurses must assume leadership roles in designing new systems of care that demonstrate the essential value of nursing's comprehensive, integrated, health-oriented focus.

APNs in Primary Care

What is the role of the APN in primary care? Clearly, NPs and CNMs are known as expert primary care providers who have accumulated a several-decade history of cost-effective, quality care (OTA, 1986). These APNs enact a unique scope of practice that perfectly integrates nursing and medical aspects of care. Through a comprehensive model of practice, they provide a holistic blend of care and cure services to clients.

Another APN is the clinical nurse specialist (CNS). There are important issues regarding the role of the clinical nurse specialist in primary care (Mirr, 1993). First, most CNSs are educated for specialty practice with acutely ill patients who often are identified by their medical diagnosis or body system (e.g., cardiovascular, renal, neurological). Although these CNSs are APNs, they are not educated to provide primary care, which is a unique specialty. Many of them are returning to graduate programs to become proficient in primary care. Second, there is a new movement to prepare CNSs to expand their scope of practice to include medical management. These CNSs will be called acute care NPs, and their expertise will be in acute care, not primary care.

It is important to emphasize that only NPs who are educated in primary care should provide primary care. But where does primary care end and acute care begin? Should the type of care be determined by the setting in which it is delivered, or is this too narrow a definition? At what point does a patient require different nursing expertise, and how is this transition managed? These issues regarding CNSs or acute care NPs and their interface with the primary care NP will continue to require nursing's attention.

NPs have always valued their holistic, comprehensive approach to patient care. Will it be cost-effective for NPs to deliver holistic, comprehensive care one patient at a time, or must we develop creative new systems of care that use a variety of health personnel? For example, some women's clinics use LVNs and health counselors to provide basic health education to the patient. The NP conducts a clinical exam and prescribes necessary treatment. A study of patient satisfaction conducted in this system found that patients were satisfied and did not feel that their care was fragmented. NPs in this system, however, reported that they felt uncomfortable when they did not provide all the essential patient education themselves (Langdon, 1990).

An explosion of demand for primary care services is expected with health care reform. Patients new to the system and current users will begin to access basic primary care services as never before. Who will provide care to these people? How can the NP sustain a holistic approach to care? Do data exist about the outcomes of this approach to care that justify the greater use of time and resources? Are there other ways to create holistic systems of care that take full advantage of support personnel while preserving the NP role for the level of care that only the NP can provide? Or will the NP adopt a more medical-model style of care, seeing patients more rapidly and focusing on "complaint-based" care? Can technology, specifically telematics and informatics, save wasted or less productive time so that comprehensive approaches to care can be maintained? Will NPs become increasingly disenchanted if they are not able to implement the model of care they value?

NPs must become involved in designing new systems of care that provide a comprehensive yet cost-effective model of patient care that does not require the NP to implement every aspect of care. A key issue for NPs will be to determine what aspects of care can and should be delegated to others. They must negotiate the resources required for creative NP models of care that are compatible with the goals and budget of the organization in which they practice. NPs will be challenged because they will provide the highest level of expertise in most care settings, yet because they are nurses, they may have self-expectations or be expected by others to enact a variety of responsibilities that could be effectively entrusted to an RN. The question may not be whether an NP *could* be responsible for an activity but whether she *should* be—is it in the best interests of the organization or the patient?

Many questions will be raised regarding the NP-RN role interface. As mentioned earlier, what are the boundaries between clinical practice for the APN and for the RN? For example, who can provide EPSDT screening exams more cost-effectively for Medicaid clients—NPs or RNs? Who should provide general health assessments for families and individuals? Differentiation of the APN and RN roles will be critical in a reformed system so that the APN is used most effectively and efficiently.

An important issue regarding the APN role is whether this nurse functions under the auspices of nursing or medical administration. Although it is believed that the majority of APNs function in nursing positions at present, there is a growing trend for medical departments to employ NPs and to bill third-party payers for their services. There is a concern that NPs who report to a medical administration may be seen largely as physician substitutes and be expected to enact a purely medical model role. Nursing administration oversight is not without problems either. For example, some NPs who function in a nursing line report that nurse administrators do not always understand the broad scope of practice or some of the unique issues faced by NPs. In smaller primary care organizations, master's-prepared NPs may be more highly educated than the nurse administrator. In fact, NPs may be responsible for administration of smaller primary care sites.

APNs will continue to evolve new systems of care, as they have with ambulatory nursing centers and community nursing organizations. Indeed, these nursing systems provide a rich range of health services extending from illness care to case management, to health education and health promotion for groups and individuals. APNs will continue to move from the shadow of physician colleagues and be recognized increasingly for the quality care they provide and the outcomes they achieve. They are the preferred providers for primary care, with their broad-based assessment skills, comprehensive focus, expertise in interpersonal therapeutics, and orientation to health and disease prevention.

Nurse Administrator Roles in Primary Care

There are several recent movements in the health industry toward the rapid development of large managed-care systems (Eckholm, 1993). These systems emphasize ambulatory rather than inpatient care, primary rather than specialty services, and management through a continuum of care rather than fragmented, episodic care. Although these new systems of care will present formidable challenges, these can be effectively addressed by expert nurse administrators (NAs).

NAs will need to assume key roles and responsibilities in designing and overseeing these systems of care, which will have a different set of priorities than current systems. For example, in a vertically integrated system of care (e.g., hospital, clinic network, home health agency, and cancer treatment center), administrators must be skilled at coordinating patient care across various units so that patients and families experience a seamless delivery system. Organizations will prioritize their services to prevent disease and to reduce drastically the need for costly hospitalization. NAs will need to be involved in what has been referred to as "upside-down thinking," in which everything is the opposite from what it was before. For example, when patients were hospitalized before, hospitals received money for their care. In a managed-care system with a capitated approach, the hospitalization of a patient will cost the system, not a third-party payer. The way to make money, or at least to reduce costs, is to keep patients out of the hospital. This new imperative means that primary care services will drive the system. Systems that achieve success in promoting health, maintaining health, preventing disease, or identifying problems in their early stages will survive. Those systems that engage in business as usual will fail.

Do we know enough to be effective in new systems of care? Do we have evidence of which approaches and which personnel are most effective? HMOs have provided years of data about how to reduce health care costs, but they have accomplished this largely through selective enrollment of working people—those people who are healthy enough to be employed and who are likely to have had access to health care for several years. What knowledge base do we have in providing care to underserved and vulnerable groups? What do we understand about case management, outreach services, follow-up, and case finding? How does one organize a system to do this, and what services are essential? Since the 1960s, the federal government has funded community health centers that are located in underserved areas serving vulnerable populations. The rich database resulting from decades of experience with these primary care models must be carefully explored and key lessons extracted. Administrators do not have all the answers needed to move forward with ease into a reformed health care system, but nurses and NAs have the critical knowledge and skills to create, implement, and manage the systems we need.

What specific knowledge and skills do NAs need to enhance their effectiveness in primary care environments? First of all, NAs must bring generic leadership and administrative skills that apply regardless of the practice setting. Possible new skill areas for NAs include facilitating the development of teams of professionals who are each willing to expand their boundaries and learn new roles and responsibilities, providing leadership in the development and testing of new models and systems of care, involving community members as partners in the process of developing and managing a primary care system, creating and sustaining a culturally competent staff and a culturally sensitive system, fostering networks with other agencies and programs with whom care will have to be coordinated, defining essential system variables and community variables that will form an epidemiologic database necessary for the planning and evaluation of primary care, and making hard decisions that balance cost issues with quality-of-care issues.

It will be particularly important for NAs to demonstrate the ability to take risks in relatively unknown areas and to tolerate ambiguity as new programs are developed and tested. They must be willing, even eager, to promote the exploration of new roles within their system. Most of all, they must be open to the development and support of creative approaches and bold innovations. They must communicate clearly and without delay to their colleagues in nursing education about the type of professionals and skills needed in the new settings.

I challenge each NA who will assume responsibility for administration of primary care settings to become acquainted with this area of practice. Spend 1 week immersed in a primary care setting: Spend time with the NP; do not just discuss her role, but shadow her as she sees patients. Begin to understand the truly wonderful scope of practice she provides. Go on home visits with the RN or community worker to develop a firsthand experience in the community. Attend a community meeting and learn about the different approaches and different rhythms that community members bring to decision making. Spend time in the local laundromat observing community life. Talk to school administrators, public health colleagues, and community members about their perspectives of community needs and how they would like to be involved. NAs cannot provide creative leadership if they do not understand the community they serve and the daily lives of their staff. NAs must create and sustain the new partnerships that will be vital to a reformed health system.

REFERENCES

Agency for Health Care Policy and Research. (1993). *Putting research into practice: Report of the Task Force on Building Capacity for Research in Primary Care* (AHCPR Pub. No. 94-0062). Washington, DC: Government Printing Office.

Allan, J., & Hall, B. (1988). Challenging the focus on technology: A critique of the medical model in a changing health care system. *Advances in Nursing Science, 10*(3), 22-34.

American Nurses Association. (1991a). *Advanced practice nurses: An innovation for primary care: A fact sheet.* Washington, DC: Author.

American Nurses Association. (1991b). *Nursing's agenda for health care reform.* Washington, DC: Author.

Colwill, J. (1992). Where have all the primary care applicants gone? *New England Journal of Medicine, 326,* 387-393.

Council on Graduate Medical Education. (1992, October). *Third report: Improving access to health care through physician workforce reform.* Washington, DC: U.S. Dept. of Health and Human Services.

Courtney, R. (1995). Community partnership primary care: A new paradigm for primary care. *Public Health Nursing, 12*(6), 366-373.

Eckholm, E. (Ed.). (1993). *Solving America's health-care crisis.* New York: Random House.

Frenk, J., Gonzalez-Block, M., & Alvarez-Manilla, J. (1990). First contact, simplified technology, or risk anticipation: Defining primary health care. *Academic Medicine, 65,* 677-681.

Fuchs, V. (1986). *The health economy.* Cambridge, MA: Harvard University Press.

Health Resources and Services Administration. (1994). *The registered nurse population: Findings from the National Sample Survey of Registered Nurses, March 1992.* Washington, DC: Government Printing Office.

Institute of Medicine. (1978). *A manpower policy for primary health care* (IOM Publication 78-02). Washington, DC: National Academies of Science.

Institute of Medicine. (1984). *Community-oriented primary care: A practical assessment* (Vols. 1 & 2). Washington, DC: National Academy Press.

Institute of Medicine. (1994). *Defining primary care: An interim report.* Washington, DC: National Academies of Science.

Langdon, J. (1990). *Descriptive analysis of a nurse practitioner managed system of prenatal care.* Unpublished master's thesis, University of Texas at Arlington.

Meyer, J. A., & Silow-Carroll, S. (Eds.). (1993). *Building blocks for change: How health care affects our future.* Reston, VA: Economic and Social Research Institute.

Millis, J. S. (1966). *The graduate education of physicians: Report of the Citizens Commission on Graduate Medical Education.* Chicago: American Medical Association.

Mirr, M. (1993). Advanced clinical practice: A reconceptualized role. *AACN Clinical Issues in Critical Care Nursing, 4,* 599-602.

Nutting, P. A. (1987). Introduction. In P. A. Nutting (Ed.), *Community-oriented primary care: From principle to practice* (HRSA Publication No. HRS-A-PE 86-1, pp. xv-xxvii). Washington, DC: Government Printing Office.

Office of Technology Assessment. (1986, December). *Nurse practitioners, physician assistants, and certified nurse-midwives: A policy analysis* (Health Technology Case Study 37, OTA-HCS-37). Washington, DC: Government Printing Office.

Petersdorf, R. G. (1993). Graduate medical education: A lesson in nongovernance. In T. Q. Morris (Ed.), *Proceedings of a conference, Taking Charge of GME: To Meet the Nation's Needs in the 21st Century* (pp. 181-202). New York: Josiah Macy, Jr. Foundation.

Safriet, B. (1992). Health care dollars and regulatory sense: The role of advanced practice nursing. *Yale Journal of Regulation, 9,* 417-488.

Starfield, B. (1992). *Primary care: Concept, evaluation, and policy.* New York: Oxford University Press.

Starr, P. (1992). *The logic of health care reform.* California: Grand Rounds.

U.S. Dept. of Health, Education, and Welfare. (1971). *Secretary's Committee to Study Extended Roles for Nurses: Extending the scope of nursing practice.* Washington, DC: Government Printing Office.

World Health Organization. (1978). *Primary health care.* Geneva: Author.

CHAPTER 4

Nursing-Sensitive Outcomes in Ambulatory Care

Ida M. Androwich
Sheila A. Haas

Despite rapidly evolving care delivery models in ambulatory care and a dramatic increase in the use of the ambulatory setting for care delivery, there is little in the nursing literature regarding definition and measurement of nurse-sensitive outcomes in ambulatory care. Yet given the nature of ambulatory care patient encounters and the current emphasis on cost containment, the selecting and measuring nursing-sensitive outcomes in ambulatory care are imperative. This chapter delineates areas to be considered in specifying distinctive nursing-sensitive outcomes in ambulatory care— here defined as interventions provided in situations in which client-nurse contact is 23 hours or less during an episode of care. A systems approach to conceptualizing ambulatory care outcomes is outlined and developed. Distinctive characteristics of the ambulatory care setting and ambulatory nursing practice are outlined along with their potential impact on outcome definition and measurement. Issues associated with defining, developing, and measuring nursing-sensitive ambulatory outcomes are discussed, and possible solutions are presented.

Defining and measuring nursing-sensitive outcomes for inpatient settings has been an ongoing challenge (Jennings, 1991; Lower & Burton, 1989; Marek, 1989a, 1989b). In fact, Hegyvary (1992) concluded that the "assessment of outcomes is one of the greatest challenges in health care research. Their definitions are elusive, difficult to validate, and based on varying perspectives and world views" (p. 23). Marek (1989a, 1989b) concluded that although much work has been accomplished in nursing on outcome development, a unified framework to classify outcomes and national outcome norms are necessary. Johnson and Maas (1994) provided a comprehensive overview of the evolution of outcomes research to the present and discussed the concept of nursing-sensitive patient outcomes. Although McCormick (1991) reviewed nursing-sensitive patient outcomes in hospital settings, there is little in the nursing literature regarding definition and measurement of nursing-sensitive outcomes in ambulatory care (Miller, 1989). Yet given the nature of ambulatory care patient encounters, the number of rapidly evolving delivery models in ambulatory care, and the overall context of ambulatory care, the task of selecting and measuring nursing-sensitive outcomes in ambulatory care is not only challenging but imperative.

This chapter delineates areas to be considered in specifying distinctive nursing-sensitive ambulatory outcomes and uses a systems approach to conceptualizing these outcomes. For purposes of this chapter, ambulatory care is defined as an episode of care provided in 23 hours or less. Issues associated with defining, developing, and measuring nursing-sensitive ambulatory outcomes are examined.

STATE OF THE ART

Lack of a Unified Language for Ambulatory Nursing Practice

Ambulatory nursing practice suffers, as does all nursing, from the lack of a unified language to describe the four nursing practice elements in the Nursing Minimum Data Set (NMDS). The elements of nursing diagnosis, nursing intervention, nursing outcome, and nursing intensity must be embedded in the documentation of practice (Werley & Lang, 1988). The absence of standardized language for these elements makes it difficult to track data both within and across organizations. Numerous issues related to the adoption of such a language have been identified elsewhere (Androwich & Stoupa, 1994; Hays, Norris, Martin, & Androwich, 1994; McCloskey & Bulechek, 1994; Milholland, 1992). Nevertheless, in a climate of health care reform, with an increasing movement toward ambulatory care and a rapid acceleration in managed care, the absence of professional consensus on standardized languages must not prevent ambulatory nurses from defining and employing standard terminology to describe their practice and practice outcomes.

Nursing Minimum Data Set
in Ambulatory Settings

The need for a uniform nursing minimum data set in ambulatory care that includes the measurement of nursing outcomes was recognized several years ago by the American Academy of Ambulatory Care Nursing (AAACN; formerly the American Academy of Ambulatory Nursing Administration). In 1990, the organization convened a preconference research workshop prior to its annual meeting specifically to address the data needs of ambulatory nursing practice. In preparation for this workshop, ambulatory nursing administrators were asked to use Werley's Nursing Minimum Data Set (NMDS) collection tool (Werley, Devine, & Zorn, 1988; Werley & Lang, 1988) to document the current use of NMDS elements in ambulatory records at their institutions. Overall, the results of this exercise suggested a disappointingly low consistency in the use of Werley and Lang's (1988) four nursing elements in ambulatory care nursing documentation. In addition, when these elements were captured, they were typically recorded in a manner unique to each setting, thus providing little opportunity for cross-site comparisons. Nevertheless, the conference served to focus ambulatory nursing administrators on the importance and necessity of defining the nursing elements in ambulatory care and developing nursing databases that include diagnoses, interventions, and outcomes elements (Androwich & Phillips, 1992).

Dimensions of Nursing Work
in Ambulatory Care

Finally, the definition and specification of nursing-sensitive client outcomes in ambulatory care have been slow to develop because there has been little research reported on the dimensions of nursing work in ambulatory care. The literature is limited to single-site studies (Tighe, Fisher, Hastings, & Heller, 1985; Verran, 1981), all of which predate health care reform activities. The only national study reported to date was completed by Hackbarth, Haas, Kavanagh, and Vlasses (1995).

DEFINING AMBULATORY CARE OUTCOMES

One's perspective or worldview will influence how outcomes are defined and which outcomes are focal. For example, nursing staff in ambulatory care may be more focused on nursing-sensitive patient outcomes, whereas managers will be concerned not only with nursing-sensitive patient outcomes but also with nursing-sensitive ambulatory care outcomes and organizational outcomes in ambulatory care.

Because ambulatory care patients reside in the community and are responsible for health care decision making and provision of their own health care, the definition of *ambulatory care* given at the beginning of this chapter incorporates some aspects of home care. Rinke's (1988) definition of a health outcome in home care can thus be used as a starting point for a definition of ambulatory patient outcomes. Rinke defined a health outcome as "a measurable change in a client's state of health related to receipt of health care services" (p. 39). Four key elements in this definition merit further discussion: *measurable change, state of health, related to,* and *health care services.* With regard to *measurable change* in defining ambulatory care outcomes, should we look only at what is measurable, and should we rely only on objective measurement? Some of the most important outcomes in ambulatory care may be those that defy measurement. For example, objective measurement of quality is challenging, but subjective assessment is not. Existing instruments capture only limited characteristics of quality, which has been defined as what the client says it is and which is therefore more likely to be reflected in indirect, subjective measures (Peters, 1987). Further, Rinke's definition describes only changes as they occur to the client and does not allow for changes in family functioning. It is also problematic to assume that outcomes must be changes in status, for in some cases, a favorable outcome is *no* change in status. Nonetheless, Wilson (1993) suggested that outcomes measurement beginning with quantifiable functional and health status statistics at the point of nurse-patient contact "will alleviate the dearth of reliable patient outcome information" (p. 13).

Another crucial term in Rinke's definition is *state of health.* How *health* is defined must be explicated. Just as one's view of the provider's ability and responsibility to affect the client's health determines the scope of outcomes selected, so does one's definition of *health.* Smith (1981) gave four very distinct conceptualizations of health, each reflective of a different theoretical bias, from the highly technical medical model to the holistic eudaimonistic model. Many nurses, especially those with a commitment to primary health care, choose the latter and define *health* in its broadest sense.

The term *related to* suggests a causal relationship. This is perhaps the most challenging aspect of defining outcomes: specifying the linkages between health care services and their respective outcomes. Finally, the use of the term *health services* raises the question of how to partition the relative contributions of different health providers and their respective interventions. More specifically, how can one capture the unique contribution of nursing?

Blumberg (1986) defined outcomes as "those changes, either favorable or adverse, in the actual or potential health status of persons, groups or commu-

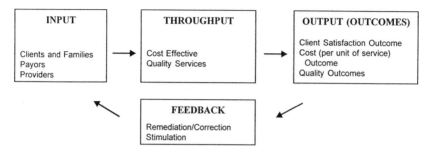

Figure 4.1. Systems Model
SOURCE: Adapted from Davis, Levine, & Sverha (1986) and Katz & Kahn (1978).

nities that can be attributed to prior or concurrent care" (p. 351). For purposes of this chapter, *nursing-sensitive ambulatory outcomes* are defined as changes in the actual or potential health status, behavior, or perceptions of individuals, families, or populations that can be attributed to nursing interventions provided in an ambulatory care setting in which client-nurse contacts may be single or intermittent contacts of 23 hours or less.

SYSTEMS APPROACH TO CONCEPTUALIZING AMBULATORY OUTCOMES

An open-systems framework (Katz & Kahn, 1978) is a useful method to organize discussion on the specification and development of measurable nursing-sensitive outcomes in ambulatory care. This framework has been used to explicate outcomes as a part of the process of delineating nursing productivity (Davis, Levine, & Sverha, 1986). Figure 4.1 illustrates the basic systems model with the four major concepts of input, throughput, output, and feedback. The term *input* is used to view some of the elements that must be considered in an ambulatory care system. The term *throughput* encompasses the services delivered, particularly those provided by nurses, in response to the inputs coming into the system. *Output* or outcomes are the projected results of the services or interventions provided as throughput. Finally, *feedback* is information gained from outcomes that may be used to influence the recycling of input into and through the ambulatory care system.

Inputs

There are multiple inputs in an ambulatory care system. Three major ones are the client, the payers, and the providers.

The following are some characteristics of the client (or the client and family) that exist in or are unique to ambulatory care:

- The client resides in the community.
- The client has some level of wellness.
- The client cannot be assumed to be only an individual because the family constellation must be considered and may in fact be responsible for day-to-day care.
- The client is in an ambulatory setting for only a brief period of time, ranging from a few minutes up to 23 hours.
- The client's visits are spaced at intervals—for example, over weeks, months, or years.
- The client is relatively autonomous in the decision making to seek care and/or to comply with care prescriptions.
- The client is typically seeking primary health care services, traditionally provided by a physician, whereas in the hospital setting the need for nursing care is a major reason for hospitalization.

The following are some characteristics of the payer:

- The payer's coverage for service is influenced by the payer's definition of health and illness.
- The payer's reimbursement for services may be fee for service, capitation based, or a modification of the above methods.
- The payer exerts varying levels of influence on the provider and provider care decisions.
- The payer demands maximum quality for least cost.
- Payers vary in levels of sophistication in tracking outcomes.

The following are some characteristics of the provider:

- The provider in the ambulatory care encounter has varying levels of professional preparation and skills (e.g., RN, MD, nurse practitioner, clinical specialist, LPN, technician or assistive worker).
- The type of agency varies (e.g., free-standing center, academic health center, physician group practice, military setting, HMO, small private practice).
- The provider may be an employee or self-employed.
- The provider may be working under fee for service or managed care or some variation of the two.

Thus there are many client "types," ranging from the person seen once by the MD and never seen by the nurse, to the MD-RN "shared" practice client, to the client whose sole provider is the RN.

Throughput

Nursing diagnoses and interventions can be viewed as one form of throughput, or nursing work or health care services offered a client. Throughput is assumed to be responsive to client and payer characteristics.

The following are some characteristics of nursing work in ambulatory care:

- Nursing assessment, diagnosis, and planning are rapid.
- The nurse often does not provide direct care to the client or family.
- Many nursing interventions, such as assessment, teaching, and follow-up, are done on the patient's behalf but not in direct or face-to-face contact with the client and are often done by phone.
- The nurse may initiate care via teaching or demonstrations, but follow-up may be by phone or at the next client visit.
- Only a portion of the care provided in ambulatory care is provided by the nurse. Physicians and other health care providers are significant players in the ambulatory patient encounter.

The dimensions of the nurse role in ambulatory care are evolving, but dimensions that have consistently appeared in the literature are teaching, advocacy, and care coordination (Hackbarth et al., 1995; Tighe et al., 1985; Verran, 1981).

Output

To definitively state (to the extent that we are able) outcomes that are related to nursing care, there should be a link from nursing assessment, diagnosis, planning, and interventions to outcomes. Some of the outcomes that might be identified, measured, and tracked are individual patient outcomes, such as patient satisfaction; aggregate patient outcomes; programmatic outcomes; and system outcomes.

Examples of individual patient outcomes that should result from interventions that are a part of major dimensions of the ambulatory nursing role are client learning, compliance with treatment regime, and client satisfaction. Some aggregated client outcomes of interest are rates of complications from a specific disease or condition or numbers of hospital admissions in a specific patient population. Programmatic outcomes for a woman's health program could include percentage of women receiving mammograms or Pap smears. System outcomes of interest could include costs of operation (per visit/by unit) and staff satisfaction.

Feedback

Information feedback that will continue to influence the ambulatory system includes client and staff responses that result from experiences of satisfaction with system functioning. Clients will in all likelihood exercise more and more decision making in their choice to continue with care in any system on the basis of satisfaction with the care provided. Health care professionals will also make choices regarding continuation of employment in a system on the basis of experiences of job satisfaction. The nurse is often pivotal in maintaining client and health care team satisfaction.

SPECIFYING DISTINCTIVE
OUTCOMES IN AMBULATORY CARE

Specification of nursing-sensitive outcomes in ambulatory care must be tied to characteristics of customers or clients of ambulatory systems (inputs) and nursing role dimensions (throughputs) that specifically respond to the requirements of customers. There is longitudinal agreement (Hackbarth et al., 1995; Tighe et al., 1985; Verran, 1981) that one of the major dimensions of the ambulatory nursing role is teaching. Therefore teaching outcomes need to be specified that capture the relationship of outcomes to teaching interventions and demonstrate the impact of nursing. The same follows for other major ambulatory nursing role dimensions such as advocacy and care coordination (Hackbarth et al., 1995).

Marek (1989b) summarized the earlier outcome classification efforts reported in the literature. Such efforts represent varying methods of classifying outcomes, ranging from diagnosis to resource use to rehabilitation status. Some have been used primarily in specific settings, such as home care. In the absence of an alternative, commonly accepted nursing-sensitive outcome classification framework for outcomes, Benson's (1992) ambulatory care outcomes categories can be useful.

Benson's (1992) classification contains the following four categories of ambulatory outcomes: (a) disease-specific outcomes, (b) general health outcomes, (c) patient performance outcomes, and (d) patient satisfaction outcomes. His work is designed to be responsive to clients being cared for in ambulatory systems. For example, Benson's *patient performance outcomes* of patient understanding and patient compliance can be used to define the outcomes of teaching implemented by the nurse. *Patient satisfaction* as an outcome can be related to nursing interventions that are undertaken as part of the advocate and care coordinator dimensions. *General health outcomes* call attention to the need to track the effect of health provider activities in the area of health promotion. Ambulatory care is not limited to illness care. Nursing-sensitive patient outcomes must be specified so that nursing work in the area of health promotion and disease prevention can be tracked. Finally, Benson's delineation of the concept of *patient satisfaction,* with its three dimensions of amenities of care, art of care, and results of care, is an example of a framework that could be used for development of nursing-sensitive ambulatory outcomes in a specific area. This type of outcome framework would provide a more complete picture of patient satisfaction and yield specific feedback information that could influence clients' continued use of ambulatory services. On the basis of the literature reviewed, a number of issues need to be addressed if a system of nursing-sensitive patient outcomes is to be developed.

Identification Issues

The first issue in identifying distinctive nursing-sensitive outcomes in ambulatory care continues to be distinguishing the processes over which nursing maintains dominion so that data generated can then support a causal link between nursing diagnoses, nursing intervention, and specified outcomes. In ambulatory care, nursing inputs may be limited. Nursing often does not provide extensive direct care, nor is it necessarily the primary source of care. Therefore, in areas where nursing care is provided—for example, in the diagnosis of knowledge deficit and the intervention of teaching-learning—documentation formats that will trigger appropriate documentation of the nursing care must be used. Routine use of such formats, especially if they are automated, will allow for tracking and aggregation of the data relevant to nursing outcomes.

Another identification issue involves differentiating the actual outcome from the expected impact of the outcome. This issue is a challenge in developing *any* outcomes classification. If one can specify the expected impact, this will assist in determining outcomes that are high priority in terms of cost or quality of life or based upon other criteria of importance to customers served. Again, automated documentation systems should markedly increase the specification and tracking of nursing-sensitive outcomes.

The relative importance placed on specific outcomes cannot be divorced from the payment system in place. For example, under a fee-for-service system, there is little motivation to reduce or limit the number of visits, whereas in managed care or with capitated systems, there is a clear incentive to deliver care effectively in the lowest number of visits. Outcomes specified and tracked will tend to be the ones valued by the payment system.

A third issue involves the temporal occurrence or "when" question. When is it realistic to expect an outcome? For example, when can you expect that clients will understand teaching about their disease process? Ambulatory care client encounters are typically distributed over varying periods of time. There may be clusters of visits for a specific problem or visits at specified intervals over weeks, months, or years for routine chronic problems. When visits are frequent for an acute circumscribed problem, it may be easier to identify and measure outcomes than when problems are chronic and visits infrequent. With a large span of time between visits, and without appropriate measures, the nurse may not see the patient or know when (or if) an outcome has occurred. Furthermore, because of the distributive nature of ambulatory care, the concern is not for just one positive outcome within a designated period of time, but for duration and consistency of outcomes over time. Yet to determine the appropriate threshold for a given outcome, or the "how many," a database is needed. Unfortunately, there are few such historical databases in ambulatory care, and we have little experience with tracking nursing-sensitive outcomes and specifying threshold. Nor do we know how to deal with risk adjustment, or taking into account those clinical or patient characteristics that can independently affect the likelihood of a given outcome (Iezzoni, 1992).

In addition to the usual dimensions of risk, such as age, clinical stability, health status, attitudes, and preferences, other methodological considerations that influence risk adjustment are unit of analysis and time frame (Iezzoni, 1992). The unit-of-analysis issue refers to data that are collected at an individual level but are to be used in the aggregate. This requires that the measurement method be structured in advance to accommodate aggregation for unit-level analysis (Hays et al., 1994; Whiting-O'Keffe, Henke, & Simbourg, 1984).

Salmon (1992) urged nursing to "count what counts." Yet how to choose what counts involves, first, consideration of the payer method, in that a fee-for-service method will value different outcomes than a capitation method. For example, in a managed-care environment, the number of ER or office visits that are avoided through the use of advice or triage by nurses is valued. Second, it should be recognized that most automated information systems are driven primarily by the need to capture financial data. Consequently nursing-sensitive ambulatory outcomes that are selected for measurement should correlate with fiscal information to document the effectiveness of clinical nursing practice. It is incumbent on nursing to ensure that the appropriate information is collected in a manner that can be aggregated and used to demonstrate nursing's value.

From this discussion, we can derive criteria for the identification of significant outcomes:

- A linkage or relationship exists between the outcome and nursing interventions.
- The outcome is valued by significant customers.
- Evidence exists of the outcome.
- Evidence can be easily tracked and aggregated.
- Aggregated data have the potential to demonstrate the unique contribution of nursing.

MEASURING OUTCOMES

No matter how well defined and specified the outcomes, if they cannot be accurately and reliably measured, they are of little value as feedback for informing future ambulatory care nursing practices. Measuring outcomes in ambulatory care engenders the same measurement issues that are encountered in other settings plus some that are unique to ambulatory care.

To capture an outcome and its cause(s) accurately, a theory or conceptual framework that both explains the construct (outcome) and its linkages and assists in the development of measurement methods that are consistent with the construct definition can be helpful. It might be argued that existing nursing theories or frameworks could be used; however, many of the nursing frameworks assume a constant nurse-patient relationship, with the nurse as care provider or supervisor of care. In ambulatory care, as has been discussed, the nurse may not be the major provider of care but may assume a coordinator role. The client is in charge. Therefore interventions may be more likely to be influenced by client variables.

In addition, the time lag between nursing interventions in ambulatory care introduces many alternative explanations such as history or maturation for changes in the outcomes that have little to do with the nursing intervention. Development of causal models that include specification of potential alternative explanatory variables is needed so that such variables can be measured whenever possible. This naturally increases the complexity of the causal model and the measurement methods.

The simple Problem → Intervention → Outcome causal chain would consequently be enhanced by specification of inputs—for example, client variables, such as demographic, disease specific, or self-care ability; provider variables, such as education, experience, or consistency of interaction with client; and payer variables, such as type of reimbursement method. In addition, unit or organizational variables could modify both problem identification and intervention, as well as the relationship between problem and intervention or intervention and outcome. There is also the potential for interactions between the above-mentioned intervening variables and time and intensity, and finally there is the issue of timing of data collection. Outcome measurement can be more complicated in ambulatory care because encounters are frequently brief and irregularly spaced at varying intervals.

Measurement of outcomes can be overwhelmingly complex if one tries to deal with all the issues of construct, internal, and external validity. A reasonable starting point is the specification and development of outcome measures and readily identifiable intervening and proxy variables. Qualitative methods should also be considered as a way to identify, delineate, and verify additional intervening variables.

Another measurement issue is that of quantitative scale sensitivity. When outcomes are to be measured over time, scales on instruments must have a sufficient range to pick up subtle changes over time. Four- or five-item Likert-type scales do not usually have sufficient breadth to capture change over time. This also requires that the researcher time the administration of instruments to fit with expected time lines of changes in outcomes.

Decisions made concerning when to measure an outcome and how to define the encounter or the episode of care under review (for which the outcome is to be measured) will influence both the selection of the indicators and the results of the measurement. In addition, statistical methods such as time-series analysis may be necessary to fully accommodate events occurring at varying intervals over time.

Measurement of nursing-sensitive outcomes assumes identification and definition of the full range of dimensions of nursing work and the nursing interventions that are a part of each dimension. There is a growing body of qualitative research that speaks of the "invisible" work of nurses (Jacques, 1993). Given the coordinating/integrating activities of ambulatory care nurses, one can speculate that this invisible work may be a major dimension of nursing work in ambulatory care. Theoretical frameworks and qualitative methods must be explored and used to make visible all dimensions of nursing work in ambulatory care so that all nursing diagnoses and interventions are available and used to explain outcomes achieved in ambulatory care.

A final measurement issue relates to the number of co-providers of care in the ambulatory encounter. Clearly, nursing is most interested in the identification and measurement of nursing-sensitive patient outcomes. Yet the specification of relative contributions of nursing when multiple providers interact and contribute to care becomes exceedingly complex. An example of this might be in a clinic area where the nurse determines the patient flow, organizes the encounter, including the history and intake process, selects the audiovisual teaching methods and materials, and prepares instruction and question-and-answer sheets for the patient to take home but does not actually interact with each individual patient. What is the nurse's contribution to the outcome(s) in this scenario?

RECOMMENDATIONS

As outcomes for ambulatory care nursing are specified and measured, it will be important to balance the value of using "industry standard" or "best practices" outcome measures with a recognition of the uniqueness of ambulatory care and the impact that individual practice settings will have on outcome specification and measurement.

Identification of Ambulatory Care Data Elements and Development of Databases

Large, computerized databases are needed that can provide comparative, easily obtainable information across ambulatory settings. With the proliferation of automated clinical information systems, it is likely that most of this data capture will be automated. But whether clinical data are captured electronically or extracted from the paper-based health record, numerous reliability and validity concerns require attention.

The National Library of Medicine (NLM) has identified the need for a Unified Medical Language System (National Library of Medicine, 1993) and has incorporated nationally recognized nursing classifications such as the North American Nursing Diagnosis Association's (NANDA's) list of nursing diagnoses, Iowa's Nursing Intervention Classification (NIC), the Omaha system, and Saba's Home Care Classification in their system. The American Nurses Association also currently supports the above four nursing classification systems. Testing the implementation and utility of these and future systems in ambulatory care must be a priority. As nursing moves toward standardizing the terminology used to describe nursing practice, cross-setting and cross-institutional comparisons will be possible.

Critical Pathways

On the basis of the recommendations of the AAACN's NMDS preconference (Androwich & Phillips, 1992), we strongly recommend that measurement of outcomes be accomplished on a routine basis via automated documentation formats. One way to accomplish this in ambulatory care is to develop critical pathways for chronic client populations. Time-centered care plans or critical pathways with time lines and critical process and outcome indicators may be designed and used as standards of care and to provide feedback on ambulatory nursing practice. Then documentation formats can be easily developed and be a part of routine care.

Critical pathways for chronic populations such as clients with diabetes, chronic obstructive lung disease, or oncology offer even greater opportunities for a return on the investment of time and energy than for populations in inpatient settings. In integrated care networks, the ambulatory setting's timed care plans or care maps can go with the client into the hospital for acute episodes of the disease and should help expedite that experience. This type of efficiency is increasingly important in capitated programs.

The creation of time-centered care plans with designated process and outcome indicators may appear to be a formidable task. However, it becomes feasible if the following suggestions are considered.

1. Start with the mission of the ambulatory care organization.
   a. Which client populations are served?
   b. Which client subgroups use high levels of resources?
   c. Which client subgroups are considered vulnerable or are targeted for added attention?
2. Examine the model of health operative in the organization.
   a. Is there one consistently and strongly held model such as the clinical model, or is there an eclectic mix of models?
   b. The care map and indicators must mesh with the model of health that is operative.
3. Nursing indicators should be reflective of typical practice in the organization and consistent with the mission and the model of health, as well as with professional standards such as the AAACN Standards (1993).

Incorporation of Primary Prevention and Health Promotion

Standards of care in ambulatory settings should routinely contain expectations regarding health promotion and disease prevention. The move to community and ambulatory care settings is concomitant with the recognition of the client's right to self-determination and the value of primary health care and prevention. One way to guarantee that institutional standards and their correlated process and outcome indicators are congruent with national norms is to use national initiatives such as the *Healthy People 2000* objectives (U.S. Dept. of Health and Human Services, 1990) to guide the development of standards and indicators. Once developed, such standards and indicators can be embedded in documentation formats. For example, currently most ambulatory organizations have standards regarding immunizations and mammograms. Table 4.1 offers process and outcome indicators that could be used in pediatric health promotion in addition to the standard indicators on immunizations. Table 4.2 offers process and outcome indicators for routine health promotion care for women that focus on breast cancer prevention.

It is important to note that most of the *Healthy People 2000* objectives are initiatives that are within the scope of independent nursing practice. Furthermore, in our cost- and quality-conscious health environment, particularly in

TABLE 4.1   Selected Ambulatory Care Process and Outcome Measures for Pediatric
            Clients

Process Indicators	Outcome Indicators
Parents are provided with classes/materials regarding age-specific nutrition.	Parents understand children's nutritional needs. Children's weight is within normal limits for age and build. Parents use resources to meet nutritional needs.
Parents are provided with teaching and materials regarding accidental injuries.	Parents demonstrate understanding of providing a safe environment for children. Incidence of preventable injury is less than the national/regional average.
Parents are provided information regarding violence to children.	Parents demonstrate an understanding of causes and measure to prevent violence to children.
Cases of child abuse do not go undetected.	Children are assessed for signs of abuse.

SOURCE: Adapted from U.S. Dept. of Health and Human Services (1990).

capitated payment systems, a case can be made that health promotion and disease prevention activities, practiced consistently, should decrease the cost per covered life. For example, if child safety seats are consistently used, accidental auto injuries to children should decrease.

CONCLUSION

When nursing-sensitive outcomes to be assessed in the ambulatory care setting have been identified and the indicators defined or developed and made measurable, critical support mechanisms must be present to enhance tracking and response to outcome measurement. These support mechanisms include documentation formats that are routinely used, automated patient records, quality improvement programming with dedicated resources, mechanisms for feedback to providers, and quality improvement initiatives that are developed and disseminated in response to outcome data analysis.

Despite the unique client, provider, and payer characteristics that serve as inputs in the ambulatory care setting, nursing has the opportunity and challenge to shape the direction of ambulatory nursing practice as a cost-effective, value-added source of care throughput. Careful attention to outcome definition and measurement will provide valid and reliable feedback to document the effectiveness of nursing care providers in the ambulatory care setting and ensure their continuing presence.

TABLE 4.2   Selected Ambulatory Care Process and Outcome Measures for Care of
Women

Process Indicators	Outcome Indicators
All clients view media and get materials on breast self-exam (BSE).	Clients demonstrate an understanding of how to do BSE. Clients report ___% compliance with BSE.
All clients are presented with their own risk factors R/T breast cancer.	Clients can discuss risk factors and appropriate responses.
Clients demonstrate understanding of effect of nutrition on incidence of breast cancer.	Clients demonstrate understanding of effect of nutrition on incidence of breast cancer.

SOURCE: Adapted from U.S. Dept. of Health and Human Services (1990).

REFERENCES

American Academy of Ambulatory Care Nursing Standards Revisions Task Force. (1993). *1993 edition ambulatory care nursing administration and practice standards.* Pitman, NJ: Anthony J. Jannetti.

Androwich, I., & Phillips, K. (Eds.). (1992). *The use of the Nursing Minimum Data Set in ambulatory nursing.* Pitman, NJ: Anthony J. Jannetti.

Androwich, I., & Stoupa, R. (1994). Count what counts: Information needs for nurse managers. *Seminars for Nurse Managers, 1*(2), 85-91.

Benson, D. (1992). *Measuring outcomes in ambulatory care.* Chicago: American Hospital Publishing.

Blumberg, M. S. (1986). Risk adjusting health care outcomes: A methodological review. *Medical Care Review, 43*(2), 351-393.

Davis, A., Levine, E., & Sverha, S. (1986). *The National Invitational Conference on Nursing Productivity: Proceedings.* Washington, DC: Georgetown University Hospital Nursing Department and Georgetown University School of Nursing.

Hackbarth, D., Haas, S., Kavanagh, J., & Vlasses, F. (1995). Dimensions of the staff nurse role in ambulatory care, Part I: Methodology and analysis of data on current staff nurse practice. *Nursing Economic$, 13,* 89-98.

Hays, B., Norris, J., Martin, K., & Androwich, I. (1994). Informatics issues for nursing's future. *Advances in Nursing Science, 16*(4), 71-81.

Hegyvary, S. (1992, October). Outcomes research: Integrating nursing practice into the world view. In *Patient outcomes research: Examining the effectiveness of nursing practice.* In Proceedings of the State of the Science Conference sponsored by the National Center for Nursing Research, September 11-13, 1991, NHH No. 93-3411 (pp. 17-24). Rockville, MD: U.S. Dept. of Health & Human Services.

Iezzoni, L. (1992). Risk adjustment for medical outcome studies. In M. Grady & H. Schwartz (Eds.), *Medical effectiveness research: Data methods* (DHHS/AHCPR Pub. No. 92-0056, pp. 83-97). Rockville, MD: U.S. Department of Health and Human Services.

Jacques, R. W. (1993). Untheorized dimensions of caring work: Caring as a structural practice and caring as a way of seeing. *Nursing Administration Quarterly, 17*(2), 1-10.

Jennings, B. M. (1991). Patient outcomes research: Seizing the opportunity. *Advances in Nursing Science, 14*(2), 59-72.

Johnson, M., & Maas, M. (1994). Nursing-focused patient outcomes: Challenge for the nineties. In J. McCloskey & H. Grace (Eds.), *Current issues in nursing* (4th ed., pp. 136-142). St. Louis: C. V. Mosby.

Katz, D., & Kahn, R. (1978). *The social psychology of organizations.* New York: John Wiley.

Lower, M. S., & Burton, S. (1989). Measuring the impact of nursing interventions on patient outcomes: The challenge of the 1990s. *Journal of Nursing Quality Assurance, 4*(1), 27-34.

Marek, K. D. (1989a). Developments in nursing classification: Classification of outcome measures in nursing care. In American Nurses Association (Ed.), *Classification systems for describing nursing practice* (ANA Publication No. NP-74, pp. 37-42). Kansas City, MO: American Nurses Association.

Marek, K. D. (1989b). Outcome measurement in nursing. *Journal of Nursing Quality Assurance, 4*(1), 1-9.

McCloskey, J., & Bulechek, G. (1994). Standardizing the language for nursing treatments: An overview of the issues. *Nursing Outlook, 42*(2), 56-63.

McCormick, K. (1991). Future data needs for quality of care monitoring, DRG considerations, reimbursement and outcome measurement. *Image, 23,* 29-32.

Milholland, K. (1992). Naming what we do: Nursing vocabularies and databases. *Journal of American Health Information Management Association, 63*(10), 58-61.

Miller, J. (1989). Evaluating structure, process, and outcome indicators in ambulatory care: The AMBUQUAL approach. *Journal of Nursing Quality Assurance, 4*(1), 40-47.

National Library of Medicine. (1993). *UMLS meta-thesaurus fact sheet.* Bethesda, MD: National Institute of Health.

Peters, T. (1987). *Thriving on chaos: Handbook for management revolution.* New York: Knopf.

Rinke, L. (1988). *Outcomes standards in home health: State of the art.* New York: National League for Nursing.

Salmon, M. (1992, October). *Keynote address.* Paper presented at the annual meeting of the American Public Health Association, Quad Council Public Health Nursing Special Session, Washington, DC.

Smith, J. (1981). The idea of health: A philosophical inquiry. *Advances in Nursing Science, 3*(3), 43-50.

Tighe, M. G., Fisher, S. G., Hastings, C., & Heller, B. (1985). A study of the oncology nursing role in ambulatory care. *Oncology Nursing Forum, 12*(6), 23-27.

U.S. Dept. of Health and Human Services. (1990). *Healthy people 2000: National health promotion and disease prevention objectives: Full report with commentary* (DHHS Pub. No. 91-50212). Washington, DC: Government Printing Office.

Verran, J. (1981). Delineation of ambulatory care nursing practice. *Journal of Ambulatory Care Management, 5*(4)2, 1-13.

Werley, H. H., Devine, E. C., & Zorn, C. R. (1988). *Nursing Minimum Data Set (NMDS) data collection manual.* Milwaukee: University of Wisconsin-Milwaukee, School of Nursing.

Werley, H. H., & Lang, N. M. (Eds.). (1988). *Identification of the Nursing Minimum Data Set.* New York: Springer.

Whiting-O'Keffe, Q. W., Henke, C., & Simbourg, D. (1984). Choosing the correct unit of analysis in medical experiments. *Medical Care, 2*(1), 1101-1114.

Wilson, A. (1993). The cost and quality of patient outcomes: A look at managed competition. *Nursing Administration Quarterly, 17*(4), 11-16.

CHAPTER 5

MOS SF-36:
Clinical and Administrative
Implications for Nurses

Cheryl L. Ramler
Vicki L. Kraus
Janet Pringle Specht
Marita G. Titler

Health care reform initiatives are placing increased emphasis on the measurement of patient outcomes as a means of evaluating the quality and effectiveness of health care services. Increasingly, health care organizations are establishing outcomes management systems made up of powerful databases that contain clinical information relative to patients' physiological status as well as information about outcomes of care that are meaningful to patients, such as their functional status and emotional well-being. Efforts to demonstrate accountability for these latter outcomes have resulted in a proliferation of instruments designed to measure health status from the patient perspective. The MOS SF-36 has emerged as one of the foremost health status measures, and its credibility reflects the painstaking efforts put forth to develop a short instrument that is psychometrically sound. The SF-36 was developed for use by practitioners as well as researchers, and it is rapidly being incorporated into many outcomes management systems. Its popularity mandates that nurse administrators be knowledgeable about the instrument and issues surrounding its use. This chapter describes the instrument, reviews its psychometric properties, and highlights issues of importance to clinical nurses and nurse administrators who are considering using the SF-36 to assess patient outcomes at the individual or aggregate level.

Health status measurement is a topic that has captured the interest of health services researchers for more than a decade. However, until recently, their concern and enthusiasm were not matched by those of clinicians, who were somewhat skeptical of the value of these instruments in measuring patient outcomes. Despite practitioners' reservations, the rising tide of health care reform has rapidly made health status measurement a necessary part of health care delivery. As health care costs skyrocket, payers are requiring that providers demonstrate how their health care practices influence patient outcomes. Functional health status has emerged as an important patient outcome because (a) it captures patients' perceptions of their day-to-day functioning and (b) it adds another perspective to more traditional outcomes such as adverse occurrences and physiological clinical data. For example, if a certain pharmacological therapy improves hemoglobin/hematocrit levels but at the same time produces increased fatigue, compromised mobility, and declining emotional well-being, one may question the value and purpose of this treatment from a functional perspective.

Increasingly, administrators of health care organizations such as hospitals, outpatient clinics, and HMOs are heeding Ellwood's (1988) recommendation to establish outcomes management systems for the purpose of documenting and monitoring the effectiveness and quality of care. The Medical Outcome Study Short Form, 36 questions (MOS SF-36), is a generic health status measure that is rapidly emerging as the forerunner in health status instruments being incorporated into these systems. The psychometric properties of the SF-36 are sound, it is relatively easy to administer, and standardized/normed data are available from specific patient populations. However, routinely adopting the SF-36 without thoughtful examination of the instrument and the application for which it is intended would be folly. Nurse administrators need to be cognizant of the issues surrounding the use of the SF-36 to ensure that the effectiveness of nursing practice, as well as medical practice, is reflected in this outcome measure. Can scores from individual patients be interpreted in a meaningful way so that nurses are able to use the information in their day-to-day management of the nursing care of patients? Are the health status scores sensitive and specific to the nursing care given? Are the scores useful to nurse managers and administrators in planning nursing care for groups of patients? The trend toward measuring health status as part of the routine assessment of certain patient populations mandates that nurse administrators be knowledgeable about health status instruments and the issues surrounding their use. Otherwise, instrument selection will proceed without informed input from nurses about the adequacy of these instruments in measuring the efficacy and outcomes of nursing interventions.

BACKGROUND

The MOS SF-36 is a health status instrument that has received considerable attention from researchers and clinicians because of its potential to measure accurately the physical and mental well-being of a wide variety of populations using a minimal number of items. A great deal of research and expertise has been applied in the development of this instrument. It evolved over a time span of approximately 17 years, beginning in 1974 with the Rand Health Insurance Experiment (HIE; Brook et al., 1983). The SF-36 and its precursor, the SF-20 (short form-20 items), were constructed from the long-form health status questionnaires used in the HIE study. The HIE was a federally supported randomized controlled trial undertaken to assess the effect of different insurance plans on the use of health care services and on health outcomes. It is regarded as a landmark study for outcomes measurement because it was the first time efforts were made to define and measure health status on the basis of both physiological indicators and the physical, mental, and social well-being of participants. One problem encountered by the researchers was the respondent burden associated with lengthy surveys. Some participants refused to complete the health status scales, which totaled 108 questions and took approximately 45 minutes to complete (Stewart, Hays, & Ware, 1988). This experience spurred the development of shorter, less time-consuming surveys that still provided valid, accurate measures of these concepts.

Experience with the long-form HIE scales provided the knowledge and information needed to develop shorter versions of the scales. Trade-offs are inevitable when long-form measures are abridged, but development of the SF-36 has proceeded in a very methodical manner with careful application of psychometric principles. John Ware, the principal author of the SF-36, spearheaded the development of this instrument since its inception in the Rand HIE. The intent of Ware and his colleagues was to strike a balance between time-consuming instruments that are not practical for large-scale use in clinical settings and single-item measures that sacrifice precision, reliability, and validity for pragmatism. The SF-36 became available for use in 1991 and is the result of refinements of the SF-20, a health status measure based on HIE scales, which was constructed for use in the 1986 Medical Outcomes Study (MOS; Tarlov et al., 1989). Patients who participated in the MOS study were selected from a population of adults with chronic medical conditions who were seen in their physicians' offices. Thus development of the SF-36 has proceeded on the basis of evaluations obtained from a population of ambulatory adults with chronic medical problems.

GENERAL DESCRIPTION
AND CONCEPTUAL FRAMEWORK

The SF-36 is a generic measure of health status. That is, it assesses concepts that are widely applicable, regardless of age, type, and severity of disease or treatments administered. The instrument contains eight multi-item scales that measure both physical and mental dimensions of health status: (a) physical functioning (PF), (b) role limitations due to physical health (RP), (c) bodily pain (BP), (d) general health perception (GH), (e) vitality (VT), (f) social functioning (SF), (g) role limitations due to emotional problems (RE), and (h) mental health (MH). A single item has also been included that asks respondents to rate the amount of change in their health status over the past year.

Generic health status measures provide a common denominator with which to make comparisons across diverse populations, making their application useful in clinical practice, research, health care management, and health policy analysis (Patrick & Deyo, 1989). One of the most well-known applications of the SF-36 was its use in the MOS to demonstrate the differential impact of five chronic diseases on health status (Stewart et al., 1989). The instrument has also been used to evaluate the effects of medical interventions (Katz, Larson, Phillips, Fossel, & Liang, 1992; Phillips & Lansky, 1992), compare different treatment modalities (Lansky, Butler, & Waller, 1992), and assess the health of the general population (Jenkinson, Coulter, & Wright, 1993). Outcomes management systems have incorporated the SF-36 into programs designed to monitor the health status of certain patient populations (Nerenz, Repasky, Whitehouse, & Kahkonen, 1992), and according to Ware (1993), the instrument is being used in at least 260 clinical trials to measure health status.

The SF-36 is recommended for use with persons 14 years and older and can be self-administered or administered by telephone or personal interview. Items are written in a Likert response format, and scores for the scales are obtained by summing responses for the items in each scale. Table 5.1 contains an explanation of the meaning of high and low scores for the scales, as well as the number of items in each. Each scale is scored separately, resulting in a profile of eight scores for each respondent. Although strategies are being investigated for constructing a single summary score for physical health and mental health, these procedures are not currently available (Ware, 1993). Scoring requires several steps, which Ware (1993) recommends be performed by a computer.

TABLE 5.1 Information About the SF-36 Health Status Scales

Scale	No. of Items	Meaning of Scores Low	High
Physical functioning (PF)	10	Limited a lot in performing all physical activities, including bathing or dressing, due to health	Performs all types of physical activities, including the most vigorous, without limitations due to health
Role—physical (RP)	4	Problems with work or other daily activities as a result of physical health	No problems with work or other daily activities as a result of physical health
Bodily pain (BP)	2	Very severe and extremely limiting pain	No pain or limitations due to pain
General health (GH)	5	Evaluates personal health as poor and believes it is likely to get worse	Evaluates personal health as excellent
Vitality (VT)	4	Feels tired and worn out all of the time	Feels full of pep and energy all of the time
Social functioning (SF)	2	Extreme and frequent interference with normal social activities due to physical or emotional problems	Performs normal social activities without interference due to physical or emotional problems
Role—emotional (RE)	3	Problems with work or other daily activities as a result of emotional problems	No problems with work or other daily activities as a result of emotional problems
Mental health (MH)	5	Feelings of nervousness and depression all of the time	Feels peaceful, happy, and calm all of the time
Reported health transition	1	Believes general health is much better now than 1 year ago	Believes general health is much worse now than 1 year ago

SOURCE: From "The MOS 36-Item Short-Form Health Survey (SF-36). I. Conceptual Framework and Item Selection," by J. E. Ware and C. D. Sherbourne, 1992, *Medical Care, 30*, pp. 473-483. Copyright 1992 by J. E. Ware. Adapted with permission.

The scoring procedure, as well as directions for handling missing data, is clearly outlined in a comprehensive manual describing the instrument (Ware, 1993). Permission to use the SF-36 can be obtained from the Medical Outcomes Trust, P.O. Box 1917, Boston, MA 02205.

Each of the SF-36 scales represents one or more of three broad dimensions of the concept of health: (a) behavioral functioning, (b) perceived well-being, and (c) general health perceptions (Ware, 1991). These dimensions incorporate phenomena that can be seen, as well as internal states that cannot be inferred from observable behaviors (Ware, 1991). A set of generic health concepts must include measures that reflect each of these dimensions to be considered an adequate representation of health status. The eight concepts chosen for the SF-36 were based on this criterion of comprehensiveness or content validity. However, not all important health concepts are represented in the SF-36. Health distress, family functioning, cognitive functioning, sexual functioning, sleep disorders, and symptoms/problems are several aspects of health status not included, and testing is currently under way to evaluate whether the addition of some of these concepts would add sufficient information to warrant lengthening the current instrument (Ware & Sherbourne, 1992).

In addition to meeting standards for comprehensiveness, construction of generic health status measures also requires consideration of the range of health states that need to be assessed (Ware, 1987). The health continuum encompasses disease states as well as conditions of physical and mental well-being and vitality. If scales are to be suitable for use in both sick and well populations, the items must reflect the wide variations exhibited by these groups. Historically, many scales used to measure health status contained items that measured only the negative end of the health spectrum and included few or no questions that would reflect the high levels of vitality and well-being that can be observed in the general population (Ware, 1987). This shortcoming limits the usefulness of an instrument by making it more difficult to detect population differences and changes over time within populations. It is difficult to demonstrate improvement in health status in populations that are already healthy when the instrument being used does not include items relating to exceptionally positive health conditions. The SF-36 contains three scales (general health, vitality, mental health) that are bipolar in nature and measure a very wide range of health states. High scores on these scales indicate not only that respondents are free of limitations or disability but that they rate their general health, energy level, and mental health very positively (Ware, 1993).

RELIABILITY

Instrument reliability is the consistency with which an instrument measures a given concept. Although repeated measurements never yield exactly the same results, they tend to be consistent with one another, and this consistency is referred to as *reliability* (Carmine & Zeller, 1979). The most widely used method of assessing reliability of multi-item measures is the internal consistency method, generally expressed as Cronbach's alpha, a measure of the correlation among items in the same scale. High correlations signify that the items all measure the same thing. Generally, the more items a scale contains, the higher its reliability will be. Thus achieving adequate reliability for short-form measures is challenging and requires repeated testing and revisions.

Reliability is important because it affects the instrument's ability to detect differences between the groups or individuals being measured. The higher the reliability of an instrument, the more likely it is to detect differences between groups or individuals or changes in scores over time. Reliability also affects how confident one can be about the accuracy of a given score: that is, whether the scores reflect the true status of the individual or group on the concept being measured. The more reliable the instrument, the more likely it is that the score accurately reflects this "true status." In general, higher reliability is recommended for individual score comparisons (.90 and above) than for group comparisons (.50 to .70), particularly for serial measures obtained from individuals across time (McHorney, Ware, Rogers, Raczek, & Lu, 1992). Individual changes over time are often small and are not likely to be detected by instruments with low reliability. Data to date indicate that reliability of all the SF-36 scales makes them suitable for group comparisons across a wide variety of populations. However, with the exception of the physical functioning scale, standards for individual patient comparisons were not met, and further study is required before the SF-36 is recommended for use in making individual treatment decisions.

Internal consistency reliability has been extensively evaluated for the SF-36. Ware (1993) listed 12 studies that report Cronbach's alphas for the eight scales, and the results are quite favorable. The reliability criterion for group comparisons (.50 to .70) was easily met. Of 63 estimates reported on the eight scales, all were higher than .60, 95% were .70 or higher, and 83% were .80 or higher. In addition, Cronbach's alpha for the physical functioning scale met minimal reliability standards for individual comparisons (.90) in six of the seven studies reported. These reliability estimates are very good for short-form scales containing a minimal number of items, and significant efforts were put into evaluating and revising the scales to achieve these results. Although reliability estimates vary with different populations and need to be calculated for the group under study, the populations in these 12 studies represent fairly diverse groups and include patients visiting their physicians, individuals with a variety of chronic illnesses (diabetes, renal disease, AIDS), and individuals from the general populations in the United States and United Kingdom. Reliability

TABLE 5.2   Internal Consistency Reliability Estimates for the SF-36 Scales

	PF	RP	BP	GH	VT	SF	RE	MH
Patients discharged from community hospital, $N = 680$ (Ramler & Specht, 1992)	.95	.90	.83[a]	.87	.84	.80	.87	.84
Participants in MOS, $N = 3,445$ (McHorney, Ware, Lu, & Sherbourne, 1994)	.93	.84	.82	.78	.87	.85	.83	.90
Random sample of U.S. population, $N = 1,692$ (McHorney, Kosinski, & Ware, 1994)	.94	.89	.88	.83	.87	.63	.81	.82

a. Scores for bodily pain were obtained by a standard scoring method.

estimates from a stratified random sample of 680 patients discharged from a community hospital in the Midwest were also very satisfactory (Ramler & Specht, 1992). Table 5.2 displays these estimates, along with those obtained using data from a sample of participants in the MOS and a random sample of the U.S. population.

CONTENT VALIDITY

Validity is the extent to which an instrument exemplifies the concept it is intended to measure. Because there is not agreement about what health status is and there is no gold standard for measurement, the validity of the SF-36 has been demonstrated using techniques recommended by the American Psychological Association. These include strategies for evaluating content, construct, and criterion validity (Carmine & Zeller, 1979). In this chapter, we focus on appraisals of content and construct validity. The scales also performed well in evaluations of criterion validity, which is discussed elsewhere (Ware, 1993).

Content validity is the extent to which the instrument items adequately represent the domain of the concept being measured. As discussed above, Ware (1987) identified the standards for judging content validity or comprehensiveness of health status measures, and construction of the SF-36 was based on these standards: (a) dimensions of health that must be measured and (b) range of measurement. To assess the comprehensiveness of the SF-36 and determine if the fundamental dimensions of health are measured, the scales were compared with those included in other widely used health status measures, including the long-form measures of the MOS and HIE, the Sickness Impact Profile, the Dartmouth COOP charts, the Nottingham Health Profile, the Duke Health Profile, the Quality of Well-Being Scale, and the McMaster Health Index Questionnaire (Ware, 1993). The SF-36 compares favorably with these other forms in terms of inclusiveness, especially for a short-form scale.

Ranges of health states measured by the SF-36 scales were assessed by evaluating score distributions for the presence of floor and ceiling effects. These effects are evidenced by large numbers of respondents scoring at the highest (ceiling) or lowest (floor) points on the scale. For example, floor effects were found for the scale measuring role limitations due to physical problems (RP) and were most evident for sicker populations. A substantial number of elderly respondents, patients with congestive heart failure, and patients with complex medical and psychiatric conditions received the lowest possible score on the RP scale (McHorney, Ware, Lu, & Sherbourne, 1994). Similar findings are reported for both role disability scales (RP and RE) in a population of patients with end-stage renal disease (Kurtin, Davies, Meyer, DeGiacomo, & Kantz, 1992). Thus, in these groups, further deterioration in health status related to RP and RE would be difficult to detect because, by these scales, many respondents' health status is already at the lowest point of the health continuum.

Floor and ceiling effects are frequently the result of coarse scales that contain a minimal number of measurement levels and therefore do not provide sufficient detail to document a wide range of conditions. They are more likely to be a problem with single-item scales. There are no single-item scales in the SF-36. Data from the MOS have been used to study the pattern of responses of the total sample as well as different patient subgroups of that sample (age, gender, race, education, poverty status, medical diagnosis, and disease severity), and the findings show that floor and ceiling effects are negligible for the bipolar scales (GH, VT, and MH) but sizable for the two role disability scales (RP and RE; McHorney, Ware, et al., 1994). These two scales are the coarsest (least precise) of the eight scales, and they demonstrated significant floor and ceiling effects in the MOS sample as a whole and also in several of the patient subgroups. In addition to the floor effects described above for the RP scale, floor effects were found for the RE scale in populations of depressed patients, patients in poverty, and patients with complex medical and psychiatric conditions (McHorney, Ware, et al., 1994). The physical functioning scale is another scale that has the potential for floor effects among severely ill populations. The scale contains only one item that focuses on self-care activities, and it may be necessary to supplement it with additional items so that a more in-depth assessment is possible with severely ill groups, geriatric populations, or patients undergoing physical rehabilitation (Ware & Sherbourne, 1992).

Ceiling effects were found for both role disability scales among patients with uncomplicated medical problems. The other scale in which ceiling effects were found was the social functioning scale. These were evident in the total MOS sample as well as in relatively healthy subgroups, such as patients with hypertension and uncomplicated medical conditions. The presence of floor and ceiling effects diminishes the scales' capacity for detecting changes in health status in these populations. These effects also prevent further differentiation of health status among individuals scoring at the floor and ceiling of the scale because the scales are not precise enough to distinguish differences at these points.

The SF-36 scales were created for a study of chronically ill outpatients, and further research is needed to determine if their usefulness with these groups can be generalized to other populations, such as hospital inpatients. In a study of patients who were sicker than participants in the MOS (individuals who had previously been admitted to the medical service in two rural public hospitals), SF-20 scores obtained 6 months after baseline failed to demonstrate any change, even though one half of these individuals reported a change in their status on each scale when they were specifically asked a transition question that was not part of the SF-20 (Bindman, Keane, & Lurie, 1990). Although some of these findings are partly due to single-item scales in the SF-20, which have been improved in the SF-36, the issue of potential floor effects in sicker populations remains. Additional studies are needed that evaluate the SF-36 scales for use with inpatient populations and other severely ill groups.

CONSTRUCT VALIDITY

A great deal of effort has been applied in evaluations aimed at establishing construct validity of the SF-36. Construct validation strategies are undertaken to assess whether scale scores correspond to other measures in a manner consistent with health status theory. Theoretical assumptions about the relationships among variables are tested. For example, is it assumed that physical function will be related to severity of illness in a certain manner (e.g., as severity increases, does physical function decline?). Empirical data demonstrating this relationship would provide evidence of construct validity.

Construct validation is an ongoing process that can be approached in many different ways. Investigators sought to substantiate that the SF-36 scales measure two aspects of health, physical and mental. Physical functioning, role limitations due to physical functioning, and bodily pain were the scales presumed to be the most valid measures of physical health, and mental health and role limitations due to emotional problems were expected to measure mental health. Vitality, general health perceptions, and social functioning were thought to capture both physical and mental aspects of health. Two distinct methods were employed to assess construct validity of the SF-36: clinical tests (comparisons of known groups) and a psychometric approach (factor analysis; McHorney, Ware, & Raczek, 1993). Factor analysis to examine correlations among the eight scales confirmed the presence of two distinct health dimensions, physical and mental. Three scales demonstrated strong correlations with the physical health dimension: physical functioning, role limitations due to physical health, and bodily pain. Three scales demonstrated strong correlations with the mental health dimension: mental health, role limitations due to emotional problems, and social functioning.

For the clinical tests of validity, comparisons were made using four groups known to differ in physical or mental health status. Clinical criteria were used to classify a sample of patients who participated in the MOS as having (a) uncomplicated chronic illness, (b) serious chronic illness, (c) psychiatric disorder, or (d) both serious chronic illness and a psychiatric disorder. Using the SF-36, comparisons were made to determine which scale best differentiated groups differing in severity of medical illness and which scale was best for classifying groups differing in the presence and severity of psychiatric disorders. The physical function and mental health scales, respectively, were demonstrated to be most sensitive to physical and mental health differences. Role limitations due to physical health and general health perceptions were the other two scales that consistently differentiated groups differing in severity of medical illness. Role limitations due to emotional problems ranked second to the mental health scale for detecting psychiatric problems (McHorney et al., 1993).

Results from these validity analysis have implications for score interpretation. The physical functioning and mental health scales are relatively pure measures of physical and mental health status, respectively. An unexpected finding was that the general health perception scale also represents primarily the physical health dimension. This simplifies score interpretation (e.g., high scores on physical function can be attributed solely to sound physical health status). The two role disability scales are also primarily unidimensional but not entirely, and less confidence can be attached to inferences made about the underlying cause of these scores. Interpretation of the other scales is more ambiguous because they reflect both physical and mental health dimensions. The vitality scale was designed to tap both physical and mental health dimensions, and this was confirmed by both validity methods. Likewise, social functioning scores reflect emotional problems that hinder social function, but they are also moderately sensitive to the burden associated with physical illness. Score interpretation for these scales is confounded by the more complex nature of their underlying structure (McHorney et al., 1993).

SENSITIVITY/RESPONSIVENESS

Another criterion on which health status measures are judged is their responsiveness or sensitivity to clinical change: that is, whether the instrument can detect changes that may be small but clinically significant. This issue is of particular concern to clinicians who want to use information from health status scales to evaluate change over time. Although generic measures, such as the SF-36, provide the means for comparing health status outcomes among diverse populations, clinicians remain skeptical about their potential to detect change in outcomes that are specific to certain diseases or conditions. Many disease-specific or condition-specific instruments, such as the Arthritis Impact Measurement Scales, have been developed to measure outcomes considered most relevant for particular populations. The content of disease/condition-specific measures may be very similar to that of generic measures, but the items often contain greater detail about functions or symptoms common to that group. Patrick and Deyo (1989) described disease-specific measures as "translations of generic health status concepts into the cultural categories, vocabularies, and perspectives of different groups" (p. S228).

As expected, there are tradeoffs associated with the use of either generic or disease/condition-specific measures. Instruments designed for special populations may be more responsive to changes occurring within subjects as the result of treatment or the progression of the disease. However, they do not permit comparisons between diverse populations, and they do not reflect the combined effects of multiple health problems for patients with more than one diagnosis. Decisions about which measure to use are driven by the objectives of measurement. Nurse clinicians interested in testing the effects of nursing interventions may prefer disease/condition-specific instruments. Nurse administrators who want to use health status measures as a basis for comparing treatment programs (e.g., rehabilitation) across diverse patient populations require data from generic measures. A combined approach using both generic and specific measures has been recommended for some applications (Kantz, Harris, Levitsky, Ware, & Davies, 1992). But this methodology may necessitate the development of supplements to generic measures that are disease/condition specific so that overlap and coincident respondent burden are reduced when the two instruments are administered together. Comparison studies are needed that evaluate the relative sensitivity of the two forms of measurement in the same population. If the specific measures are no more sensitive than their generic counterparts, the latter will have broader applications.

Preliminary efforts to evaluate the specificity of the SF-36 have begun to appear in analyses of this instrument. One study compared the sensitivity and specificity of the SF-36 with those of condition-specific instruments that measured the same concepts in patients who had total knee replacements (Kantz et al., 1992). On the basis of their findings, the authors concluded that the specific measures of knee pain and role limitations due to knee problems were more sensitive instruments than the generic measure of the SF-36. However, the condition-specific measure of limitations in physical functioning was not more sensitive than the generic measure in the SF-36. In a longitudinal study of patients undergoing total hip arthroplasty, researchers compared the measurement sensitivity of the SF-36 and three other short-form measures with a longer health status instrument, the Sickness Impact Profile (SIP; Katz et al., 1992). Scales of each instrument were aggregated to create scores for three dimensions of health status: physical, psychological, and global. Although the SIP was the most sensitive psychological measure, the SF-36 was more sensitive on the physical and global dimensions.

Another study compared the precision of the SF-36 and two other short-form scales (MOS 6-Item General Health Survey and COOP poster charts) with the long-form measures from the MOS (McHorney et al., 1992). *Precision* was defined as the instrument's potential to distinguish mutually exclusive clinical groups. Patients with minor chronic medical conditions were compared with two other patient groups: (a) patients with serious chronic medical conditions and (b) patients with psychiatric disorders. The long-form measure was generally the most precise, with the SF-36 ranking second. However, for some applications the drop in precision may be small enough so that the SF-36 would be the instrument of choice because of its brevity. For example, the 5-item mental health scale of the SF-36 was 93% as precise as the 32-item long-form measure in the comparison of the two medical groups and the medical/psychiatric comparison. The one scale in which the long-form measure was clearly superior to the SF-36 was the general health perceptions scale. The SF-36 was only 72% as precise as the long-form measure in the comparison of the two medical groups and 39% as precise in the medical psychiatric comparison.

Whether the SF-36 is a sensitive measure of health status changes that are affected by nursing interventions remains to be determined. Total knee replacement and hip arthroplasty are procedures that have striking effects on health status, particularly those aspects related to physical functioning and pain. The influence of nursing interventions may be more subtle, and demonstrating these effects may require more specific instruments. For example, the SIP scales include measures of outcomes that reflect more discrete aspects of health status—for example, eating, sleep and rest, and mobility. These outcomes are the objective of many nursing interventions, and documenting their effects may be achieved more easily with some of the SIP scales. But it is also conceivable that some nursing treatments, particularly those undertaken in populations with chronic illness, such as pain control, therapeutic touch, patient teaching, crisis intervention, counseling, bowel training, and intermittent catheterization, might effect health status changes that would be reflected in changing scores on the SF-36. The SF-36 might also be sensitive to health status changes produced by nursing interventions aimed at health promotion, such as exercise programs, smoking cessation, relaxation training, and weight management. Nursing research is needed that incorporates the SF-36 as an outcome measure so that its potential for documenting nurses' contributions to the health status of nurses' clients can be evaluated. The importance of such an evaluation is underscored by the increasing use of the SF-36 as part of the routine assessment of certain patient populations. If the instrument is incorporated into outcomes measurement systems, it is important to evaluate its potential to detect the effects of nursing as well as medical interventions.

RESPONDENT BURDEN AND DATA QUALITY

One very important issue to consider when evaluating an instrument is the amount of respondent burden associated with its administration: that is, how much time and energy are required to answer the questionnaire (Ware, 1993). Refusal to participate and missing responses are two consequences associated with questionnaires that are regarded as onerous to complete. Whether an individual perceives a questionnaire as difficult is dependent not only on the characteristics of the questionnaire but also on the attributes of the individual. Questionnaires that are completed effortlessly by healthy, well-educated adults in the United States might present difficulty for sicker individuals, minorities, and those from impoverished environments. Consequently an instrument's performance must be judged in relation to the population to whom it will be administered.

In general, the evidence presented demonstrates that the SF-36 performs well with regard to patient acceptance and data completeness. Response rates are one indicator of patients' willingness to complete the SF-36, and those published have been very satisfactory. An overall response rate of 85% was achieved when the questionnaire was mailed to 235 adults with diabetes who were seen at an endocrinology clinic at Henry Ford Hospital in Detroit (Nerenz et al., 1992). Questionnaires were accompanied by cover letters from the patients' physicians, and follow-up mailings and phone calls were initiated when individuals did not respond to the mailings. When no follow-up was carried out, an overall response rate of 43% was obtained with a stratified random sample of patients 2 to 6 weeks post discharge from a community hospital in the Midwest (Ramler & Specht, 1992). Patients' reactions to completing the SF-36 were also carefully observed in a population of outpatient dialysis patients, who willingly completed the questionnaire, had no negative comments about the content, and were amenable to repeated administrations at 3-month intervals (Kurtin et al., 1992). The opscan version of the questionnaire was used in this study and required approximately 15 to 20 minutes to complete. The opscan format requires respondents to darken small ovals to designate their answers, which can then be scanned to obtain a score. A number of respondents with visual problems had difficulty reading the print, prompting investigators to make a test booklet with large print available as an option. In addition, elderly patients were unfamiliar with the format of the opscan version, and some had difficulty adequately darkening the small ovals.

The percentage of completed items is another indicator of patient acceptance and also provides information about data quality. Percentage of completed items was very high when data from the outpatient sample in the MOS ($n = $ 3,445) were evaluated (McHorney, Ware, et al., 1994). All of the scales achieved 90% or higher, with the exception of the PF scale, which was 88.3%. However, analysis of subgroups from this sample did reveal that disadvantaged groups might have more difficulty with the scales. Percentages of completed items in the scales were significantly lower for individuals with less than a high school education, black patients, and those in poverty. They were also lower for elderly patients. Even though these percentages were lower, scale scores could still be computed for over 96% of these respondents by substituting a person-specific mean, which could be computed when one half or fewer of the scale items had been answered.

As these findings demonstrate, the SF-36 is easily completed by many populations. However, some groups may have difficulty with the scales. Individuals to whom the instrument is to be self-administered must have competent reading skills, as well as be physically capable of completing an answer sheet. The elderly, the poor, individuals with minimal education, and patients with cognitive or physical impairments may require assistance. Two groups for whom the instrument would not be usable are persons who do not speak English fluently and pediatric patients. However, efforts are currently under way to translate the SF-36 for use in 15 different countries, and a United Kingdom version of the instrument has been published. In addition, a

Mexican American version has been made available for select clinical trials (Ware, 1993).

USE AND IMPLEMENTATION
OF THE SF-36 IN CLINICAL SETTINGS

Use of the SF-36 has the potential for improving individual patient outcomes if integrated into clinical practice with real-time scoring (Greenfield & Nelson, 1992; Lansky et al., 1992; Nelson & Berwick, 1989; Thier, 1992). The instrument provides an efficient method of collecting health status data that are important in the initial and ongoing assessment of patient problems and in the development of a more focused plan of care. In addition, communication between providers and patients can be enhanced through the use of this instrument. Reviewing scores with the patient opens the door for discussions of areas of concern that have not been previously disclosed (Nelson & Berwick, 1989). Data from the SF-36 bring to the provider clinically relevant information from the perspective of the patient and/or family (Deyo & Patrick, 1989; Nelson & Berwick, 1989; Thier, 1992). Previously unidentified problems may become evident: The provider may not have been aware of the extent of the decline in the patient's health status, or the patient may not have volunteered the information because of incorrectly attributing the decline to natural processes such as aging instead of potentially treatable problems. In addition, if the functional decline is out of proportion to the usual pattern with a particular condition, it suggests that the diagnosis is incorrect or that an additional undetected problem exists (Greenfield & Nelson, 1992). With the availability of improved health status data comes the opportunity to select interventions and supplemental services that are focused more specifically on the individual patient's problems (Lansky et al., 1992).

Routine measurement of health status also provides an opportunity to learn about the natural history of chronic illnesses. Typical patterns or profiles of the impact of chronic conditions on health status can be described and used for evaluating patient progress (Greenfield & Nelson, 1992). The MOS demonstrated a differential impact of disease on health status with five chronic conditions: heart disease, diabetes, hypertension, myocardial infarction, and depression. Each of these chronic problems had a unique profile of effects on physical functions, mental health, social functioning, and perceived health status (Stewart et al., 1989). Knowledge of the trajectory of health status in a particular illness enables providers to time interventions more precisely, anticipate when treatment plans need to be modified, and provide feedback to patients regarding progress (Nelson & Berwick, 1989).

Although functional health status measures offer great potential for achieving clinical goals, use of these tools remains largely untried in the clinical setting. Accrual of substantial aggregate data is needed to facilitate the application of health status data to the individual patient care situation. Individual patient scores take on meaning only when a basis for comparison has been established: that is, when one can judge how an individual's scores compare with those of others who have the same clinical problem or of the population at large. Without some frame of reference, individual scores have no meaning for clinicians. This issue emerged in an outcome assessment program when clinicians were provided with scores for individual patients but no baseline values for comparison (Lansky et al., 1992). Normative data (i.e., data drawn from representative samples of selected populations) must be collected so that clinicians have a reference for interpretation, similar to average values that are provided for laboratory tests. Normative data can be gathered from the general population, from a population of patients within one or more organizations, from patients in a specific geographic region, or from patients with a particular illness. This background information can help clinicians to judge the degree of functioning and well-being experienced by an individual relative to these groups. In addition to being compiled, the data must be readily available to providers in a clinically usable form at the point of care so that the potential impact on patient care plans and outcomes becomes a reality.

The SF-36 is one of a limited number of health status instruments for which normed data are available. Descriptive statistics based on a sample of 2,474 noninstitutionalized adults ranging from 18 to 94 are published for each of the SF-36 scales (Ware, 1993). In addition to the norms for the total sample, data are provided for male and females separately and for seven different age groups (males and females separately and combined). Norms have also been estimated for the five chronic medical conditions studied in the MOS (Ware, 1993). However, statistical adjustments have not been made for factors that might confound score interpretation (e.g., sociodemographic data, disease severity, comorbidity, and baseline functional status). Controlling for the effects of these variables is important when assessing whether a patient's scores reflect the care received or are related to factors that are beyond the control of health care providers (Greenfield & Nelson, 1992). Score interpretation is a fundamental concern of clinicians when attempting to use data from the SF-36 as part of appraisals of the effectiveness of their interventions.

The decision to monitor health status for a particular patient population requires that implementation strategies be carefully planned. If the SF-36 is to be used on a daily basis to guide the delivery of care and to monitor practice, clinician acceptance is pivotal. Substantial education is required to familiarize clinicians with the content, purpose, and application of the SF-36. In addition to being knowledgeable about the instrument itself, clinicians must also be persuaded of the value of monitoring health status and motivated to incorporate the data in the planning and evaluation of interventions. This can be accomplished only if attention is given to creating an environment that facilitates an understanding of health status measurement and supports users in their efforts to incorporate this additional information into their clinical practice. Electronic systems at the point of care must be designed to collect data, generate reports, and provide feedback in a timely manner. Ideally, health status monitoring should be integrated into routine patient care activities and perceived as an essential part of the clinical management of patients (Lansky et al., 1992).

Cost considerations must also be weighed in decisions to implement systems for routine monitoring of health status. Collecting, scoring, and analyzing data may require employment of additional personnel. In one outcomes management project involving 235 patients with diabetes mellitus, Nerenz et al. (1992) estimated that the services of a three-quarter-time project assistant were required to collect and enter information from the SF-36 and the medical record into a single database. This recommendation was based in part on a concern for data quality and the difficulties encountered when existing staff are expected to add data collecting to their current responsibilities. Equipment costs can also add to the expense of an outcomes monitoring project. To provide clinicians with prompt feedback on the results of the SF-36, Kurtin et al. (1992) purchased a processing system that included a scanner, a standard computer with SF-36 software for scoring, and a printer so that scale scores could be calculated, printed, and used by clinicians at the time of patients' dialysis session. Financing an outcomes management program presents a significant challenge, especially within the context of a provider organization. Much of the work done to date has been externally funded research, and advocates who want to expand the use of health status data to include the clinical setting will be challenged to demonstrate the value and feasibility of these projects in relation to the costs (Nerenz et al., 1992). Although costs are an issue, the possibility exists that expenditures will be more than offset by savings resulting from the use of SF-36 data. This approach could be used by nurse administrators to justify the cost.

IMPLICATIONS FOR NURSE ADMINISTRATORS

Data from the SF-36 can assist nurse administrators in identifying patient needs and planning nursing care for clinical populations served by the organization.

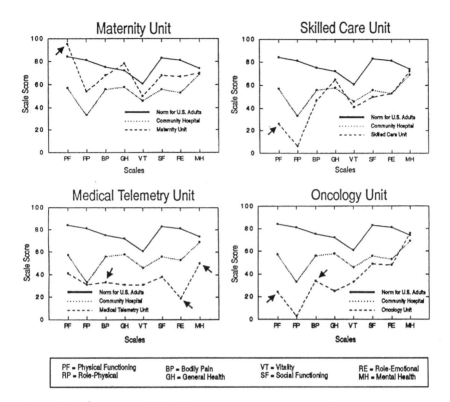

Figure 5.1. Comparison of SF-36 Mean Scale Scores for Patients Discharged From Four Units in a Midwestern Community Hospital With Mean Scale Scores for the Hospital and General U.S. Population

Profiles of scores characterizing patient populations provide information that has implications for resource allocation, personnel needs, and program development. Figure 5.1 displays score profiles from data obtained 2 to 6 weeks post discharge from patients on four units of a community hospital in the Midwest. Each diagram contains the mean scale score for the unit, the hospital, and the general U.S. population (Ware, 1993). Visual displays of the data highlight the differences among these populations and also allow unit comparisons. For example, the physical function (PF) scores for patients on the oncology and skilled care units indicate that these individuals are extremely limited in performing all physical activities and that many of them may require the assistance of home care agencies after they are discharged. Consequently resources must be allocated to meet the discharge planning needs of these groups. In addition to having discharge planning implications, low physical function scores are a gross indicator of physical care needs and may warrant more specific measures of activities of daily living. In contrast, the high scores for physical functioning on the maternity unit demonstrate the variation in scores among units, confirming the relatively healthy population expected on a maternity unit.

Several other potential needs are apparent from an examination of these score profiles. Patients on the oncology and medical telemetry units have low pain (BP) scores, indicating high levels of pain, and consequently nursing expertise in pain management would be essential for these populations. Strategies for acquiring this knowledge might include assignment of a clinical nurse specialist (CNS) for these groups and targeted educational programs for the nurses. In addition to ensuring that the knowledge base required for pain management was available within the organization, a method for evaluating the effectiveness of any pain initiative would be needed (i.e., quality assurance programs should incorporate outcome measures to assess pin management in these patient care areas). The low scores for mental health (MH) and role limitations due to emotional problems (RE) also stand out for patients on the medical telemetry unit, implying the need for particular attention to this problem or the need for specialized programming (e.g., liaison psychiatric nurse).

The SF-36 is a useful tool for quality assessment and improvement activities. As can be seen from the examples above, data from this instrument assist in the identification of problem areas and the establishment of priorities for quality improvement activities within the organization or on specific units. Scores on selected scales could be used as benchmarks for evaluation and comparison of programs and units. Prior to establishing benchmarks or standards, a database must be developed to document the normal course of an illness or response to treatment. From this information, standards or benchmarks are determined. For example, a benchmark may be established to have all total hip replacement patients attain a specific physical function score by time of discharge. Measures could continue over time after discharge through the entire continuum of care. This would require planning and coordination among a variety of health service providers. The current climate of health care reform increasingly mandates that hospitals demonstrate accountability not only for short-term treatment goals but also for long-term effects on health status. An advantage of the SF-36 is that it provides patient-based data for quality evaluation and is also an externally recognized measure (Lansky et al., 1992). This combines the important elements of patient participation in evaluation of quality and credibility to purchasers (employers, insurers, and government payers) and accrediting bodies.

SUMMARY

Changes in the American health care enterprise have placed increased demands on providers to demonstrate the impact of their services on patient outcomes, and health status has emerged as a fundamental variable in this outcomes initiative. In addition to traditional physiological data commonly measured by clinicians, increased emphasis is being placed on outcomes that are important to patients. Measurement of behavioral and psychosocial concepts indicative of physical and mental well-being has assumed greater significance as researchers and clinicians struggle to evaluate the efficacy of their interventions and as purchasers seek to identify priorities for health care expenditures. Such appraisals are incomplete without patients' reports of their functioning and well-being.

As a more comprehensive view of health has come to be accepted, efforts have focused on developing and refining instruments that are consistent with this broader perspective. Many of these instruments are very lengthy and require a great deal of time and effort to complete. In the face of health care reform, interest in shortening instruments for integration into clinical practice has emerged. The SF-36 has been constructed expressly to meet the need for shorter health status measures. Efforts to retain the psychometric properties of long-form measures from which the SF-36 scales were constructed have been largely successful. Reliability and validity have been extensively analyzed using data from the MOS, and the results are encouraging. The underlying physical and mental dimensions of health status have been confirmed by clinical comparisons of known groups and factor analysis. Reliability studies indicate that all of the scales meet standards for group comparisons. Evaluations of the instrument's sensitivity to changes in the clinical status of patients are also under way, and in some studies the short scales of the SF-36 have been shown to perform as well as condition-specific measures. In addition to having sound psychometric properties, the SF-36 has been demonstrated to be easily administered, and normative data are available for the U.S. population at large and several clinical populations. Such data are essential for clinicians to have a basis for score interpretation.

Although the psychometric properties of the SF-36 indicate that the instrument offers great potential as a health status measure, instrument selection should also be guided by the characteristics of the population to whom it will be administered and the purpose of measurement. The SF-36 was developed for use in a population of individuals with chronic illness, and many evaluations of its utility are based on studies of this group. Whether the instrument will be as useful for measuring health status in other populations requires further investigation. The role disability scales exhibited floor effects in sicker populations, and the limited number of self-care items in the physical functioning scale calls into question its usefulness in geriatric populations. Methods of administering the SF-36 also need to be carefully thought out for the elderly and other vulnerable populations, such as minorities, those in poverty, persons with minimal education, and the physically disabled. Their ability to read and comprehend the questionnaire as well as complete the form should be assessed prior to widespread adaptation of the instrument. Evaluating the utility of the SF-36 for these special populations is imperative because it is precisely these groups for whom health status assessments are needed.

One other important consideration for nurses is the sensitivity of the SF-36 to nursing interventions. Increasingly, this instrument is being adopted as part of outcomes management programs, and this provides an opportunity for nurses to incorporate SF-36 scores from outcome databases into research designed to evaluate the effectiveness of nursing interventions. Data from such research could be used to make further evaluations about the instrument's sensitivity to nursing treatments. Much work has been done to ensure that the SF-36 is psychometrically sound, and increasingly the instrument is being recognized as a premier tool for health status assessment, particularly in the clinical setting. Both nurse administrators and clinicians will encounter the instrument or data based on it with increasing frequency. Thus it is imperative to be knowledgeable about the SF-36 and also to begin evaluating its usefulness in relation to nursing practice and outcomes of concern to nurses.

REFERENCES

Bindman, A. B., Keane, D., & Lurie, N. (1990). Measuring health changes among severely ill patients: The floor phenomenon. *Medical Care, 28,* 1142-1151.

Brook, R. H., Ware, J. E., Rogers, W. H., Keeler, E. B., Davies, A. R., Donals, C. A., Goldberg, G. A., Lohr, K. N., Masthay, P. C., & Newhouse, J. P. (1983). Does free care improve adults' health? Results from a randomized controlled trial. *New England Journal of Medicine, 309,* 1526-1534.

Carmine, E. G., & Zeller, R. A. (1979). *Reliability and validity assessment.* Beverly Hills, CA: Sage.

Deyo, R. A., & Patrick, D. L. (1989). Barriers to the use of health status measures in clinical investigation, patient care, and policy research. *Medical Care, 27*(Suppl.), S254-S268.

Ellwood, P. M. (1988). Outcomes management: A technology of patient experience [Shattuck Lecture]. *New England Journal of Medicine, 318,* 1549-1556.

Greenfield, S., & Nelson, E. C. (1992). Recent developments and future issues in the use of health status assessment measures in clinical settings. *Medical Care, 30*(Suppl.), MS23-MS41.

Jenkinson, C., Coulter, A., & Wright, L. (1993). The Short Form 36 (SF-36) Health Survey Questionnaire: Normative data for adults of working age. *British Medical Journal, 306,* 1437-1440.

Kantz, M. E., Harris, W. J., Levitsky, K., Ware, J. E., & Davies, A. R. (1992). Methods for assessing condition-specific and generic functional status outcomes after total knee replacement. *Medical Care, 30*(Suppl.), MS240-MS252.

Katz, J. N., Larson, M. G., Phillips, C. B., Fossel, A. H., & Liang, M. H. (1992). Comparative measurement sensitivity of short and longer health status instruments. *Medical Care, 30,* 917-925.

Kurtin, P. S., Davies, A. D., Meyer, K. B., DeGiacomo, J. M., & Kantz, M. E. (1992). Patient-based health status measures in outpatient dialysis: Early experiences in developing an outcomes assessment program. *Medical Care, 30*(Suppl.), MS136-MS149.

Lansky, D., Butler, J. B. V., & Waller, F. T. (1992). Using health status in the hospital setting: From acute care to "outcomes management." *Medical Care, 30*(Suppl.), MS57-MS73.

McHorney, C. A., Kosinski, M., & Ware, J. E. (1994). Comparisons of the costs and quality of norms for the SF-36 Health Survey collected by mail versus telephone interview: Results from a national survey. *Medical Care, 32,* 551-567.

McHorney, C. A., Ware, J. E., Lu, J. F. R., & Sherbourne, C. D. (1994). The MOS 36-Item Short-Form Health Survey (SF-36): III. Tests of data quality, scaling assumptions, and reliability across diverse patient groups. *Medical Care, 32,* 40-66.

McHorney, C. A., Ware, J. E., & Raczek, A. E. (1993). The MOS 36-item Short-Form Health Survey (SF-36): II. Psychometric and clinical tests of validity in measuring physical and mental health constructs. *Medical Care, 31,* 247-263.

McHorney, C. A., Ware, J. E., Rogers, W., Raczek, A. E., & Lu, J. F. R. (1992). The validity and relative precision of MOS short- and long-form health status scales and Dartmouth COOP charts. *Medical Care, 30*(Suppl.), MS253-MS265.

Nelson, E. C., & Berwick, D. M. (1989). The measurement of health status in clinical practice. *Medical Care, 27*(Suppl.), S77-S90.

Nerenz, D. R., Repasky, D. P., Whitehouse, F. W., & Kahkonen, D. M. (1992). Ongoing assessment of health status in patients with diabetes mellitus. *Medical Care, 30*(Suppl.), MS112-MS123.

Patrick, D. L., & Deyo, R. A. (1989). Generic and disease-specific measures in assessing health status and quality of life. *Medical Care, 27*(Suppl.), S217-S232.

Phillips, R. C., & Lansky, D. J. (1992). Outcomes management in heart valve replacement surgery: Early experience. *Journal of Heart Valve Disease, 1,* 42-50.

Ramler, C. L., & Specht, J. P. (1992). Evaluation of patient outcomes in a Midwestern community hospital. Unpublished raw data.

Stewart, A. L., Greenfield, S., Hays, R. D., Wells, K., Rogers, W. H., Berry, S. D., McGlynn, E. A., & Ware, J. E. (1989). Functional status and well-being of patients with chronic conditions. *Journal of the American Medical Association, 262,* 907-913.

Stewart, A. L., Hays, R. D., & Ware, J. E. (1988). The MOS Short-Form General Health Survey: Reliability and validity in a patient population. *Medical Care, 26,* 724-735.

Tarlov, A. R., Ware, J. E., Greenfield, S., Nelson, E. C., Perring, E., & Zubkoff, M. (1989). The Medical Outcomes Study: An application of methods for monitoring the results of medical care. *Journal of the American Medical Association, 262,* 925-930.

Thier, S. O. (1992). Forces motivating the use of health status assessment measures in clinical settings and related clinical research. *Medical Care, 30*(Suppl.), MS15-MS22.

Ware, J. E. (1987). Standards for validating health measures: Definition and content. *Journal of Chronic Diseases, 40,* 473-480.

Ware, J. E. (1991). Conceptualizing and measuring generic health outcomes. *Cancer, 67*(Suppl.), 774-779.

Ware, J. E. (1993). *SF-36 Health Survey: Manual and interpretation guide.* Boston: Nimrod.

Ware, J. E., & Sherbourne, C. D. (1992). The MOS 36-Item Short-Form Health Survey (SF-36) I. Conceptual framework and item selection. *Medical Care, 30,* 473-481.

PART 2

Measuring and Managing Health Care Outcomes

The five chapters in Part 2 address an array of process and methodological aspects of health care outcomes measurement and management. Varied setting and approaches to outcomes evaluation and management are represented.

Spencer, Collins, and Parietti (Chapter 6) demonstrate a case management model designed to incorporate outcomes measurement. Outcomes measured are related to clients, nurses, and physicians, as well as resource utilization.

In Chapter 7, Goode et al., a team of nurse managers, offer an overview of variance tracking and analysis as a key to outcomes management by a multidisciplinary group of providers. They address the process employed, beginning with goal setting and including the feedback mechanism necessary to effective outcomes management.

Steelman (Chapter 8) offers a process for incorporating AHCPR clinical practice guidelines in outcomes management within a large teaching hospital. Specific outcomes measured in the project reported relate to impact on patients, staff, and cost.

In Chapter 9, Walters reports on a project that tested the effect of a creative staff scheduling on nurse and physician satisfaction, cost, and patient outcomes. She identifies advantages, disadvantages, and implications for subsequent innovations in staff scheduling.

The final chapter takes the reader to the world of managed care in the home health care setting. Maturen reports on the work of 10 Visiting Nurse Associations in developing clinical paths and patient outcomes measurements. She provides qualitative and quantitative evaluations of the project to date and shares how this project is evolving into a complete documentation system.

CHAPTER 6

Case Study: Facilitating the Implementation of a Case Management Model

Gale A. Spencer
Mary S. Collins
Elizabeth Parietti

This chapter presents a case study description of the development, implementation, and evaluation of a case management model in an acute care practice setting. To organize the development and implementation of the model, a 10-step framework was utilized. A discussion of the utilization of the framework for implementation of the case management model is presented. The design of the Case Management Practice Model (CMPM) emerged, and a schematic figure of the CMPM with a discussion of its components is included. Finally, outcome measurement instruments were developed to measure change in patient care utilization from the perspective of the patients, staff, nurses, and physicians.

In the fall of 1992, the clinical nurse specialists of an upstate New York community hospital were charged with developing a case management model for the delivery of care for the hospital. Because two of the clinical nurse specialists were recent graduates of the nursing master's program at an affiliating university and because the master's program had just developed and implemented the integration of case management functions within the clinical nurse specialist role courses, the faculty of the master's program were asked to serve as participants and consultants to the clinical nurse specialist (CNS) group. The faculty members and CNSs formed the Case Management Working Group (CM working group).

So that all the clinical nurse specialists would become knowledgeable about the task before them, an extensive reference list of the existing case management literature was prepared. The CM working group found that over the past 7 years, nursing literature has discussed case management in a variety of ways. It has been described as a care delivery model with the inherent potential for maximizing the quality of patient outcomes (Del Togno-Armanasco, Olivas, & Harter, 1989; Delahanty, Graves, & Hoffman, 1993; McKenzie, Torkelson, & Holt, 1989; Schull, Tosch, & Wood, 1992). Weinstein (1991) defined nursing case management within the hospital setting as a formalized multidisciplinary and integrated process for planning and delivery of a continuous plan of care for the purpose of achieving a balance among appropriate client outcomes, efficiency, quality, and cost-effectiveness. Zander (1988), however, stated that the primary goal of case management is to organize and coordinate services and resources to meet an individual's health care needs and that cost control should be a secondary objective.

The literature also supported and reinforced the CM working group's leadership role for the development and implementation of the case management practice model for care delivery. Several articles in the literature review described the clinical nurse specialist as the ideal case manager (American Nurses Association, 1988; Cronin & Maklebust, 1989; Wyers, Grove, & Pastorino, 1986). For the enactment of the CMPM project to take place, CNSs ultimately responsible for the new system of care must be part of its initial design, development, and implementation. The literature review around organizing frameworks also was a source of ideas for development and implementation of the case management system within the hospital setting (Pittman, 1991; Schull et al., 1992). One article that the CM working group found particularly helpful for organizing the development and implementation of a new model was "Ten Steps for Managing Organizational Change" (Bolton, Aydin, Popolow, & Ramseyer, 1992). The 10 steps described by Bolton et al. became the organizing framework for the project.

DEVELOPMENT OF THE MODEL

Bolton et al. (1992) stated that implementing effective system-wide change in a health care institution poses a significant challenge for those in leadership positions. They indicated that most change in a health care institution requires cooperation between two or more departments or professional groups and that managing the interdependence between the departments and groups is often forgotten. The CM working group utilized the authors' theme of "refocusing on patient care, while restructuring the organization to obtain tangible improvements in effectiveness with minimal outlay of new resources" (p. 14). The authors asserted that the 10 steps outlined in the article were essential to successful change.

IMPLEMENTATION OF THE CASE MANAGEMENT PRACTICE MODEL USING THE 10-STEP FRAMEWORK

Step 1: Define Project Goals

The project goals were identified by the hospital administration in consultation with the CNS group. The goals were (a) to develop a case management model for patient care and (b) to implement a case management model for patient care.

Step 2: Make Sure the Project Goals Are Congruent With the Organization's Strategic Plan

The CM working group was asked to develop a philosophy for the CMPM that would be congruent with the mission of the hospital, "Let the Walls Speak of Caring." The philosophy that the CM working group developed was "to promote excellence in patient care by supporting a clinical system of managed care. The delivery of quality care is enhanced by achieving patient outcomes within effective and appropriate time frames and resource utilization."

Step 3: Decide Who Will Lead the Project

The hospital administration decided that the CM working group would lead the implementation project and would serve as the case managers. The CM working group was told to select a group leader. After the group leader had been chosen and work toward development was begun, the administration decided to assign leadership responsibility to another group member to balance workloads. At this point, progress slowed down considerably. However, once the group members were able to deal with the conflict resulting from the leadership change, they were able to proceed with implementation.

Although Bolton et al. (1992) described Step 3 as defining the leadership for the project, it became clear in the CM working group that both a job description and a role description were needed to clarify the case manager role for all the constituent groups. The following description was developed:

The Nurse Case Manager assigns responsibility and accountability for the clinical management of patients in specific case groups for an episode of illness and integrates the nursing and the management processes to provide the framework for decision making within each role. The Case Manager functions in multiple collaborative roles, including manager, clinician, consultant, educator, and researcher.

The job description continues to describe in great detail the role of the nurse case manager and expectations of each of the identified roles of manager, clinician, consultant, educator, and researcher.

The CM working group also decided that a definition of the case manager's role and its relationship with other departments and professions within the hospital needed to be developed. The following definition resulted:

Clinical nursing specialists designated as Case Managers for selected patient populations[1] facilitate the implementation of managed care. In collaboration with Medicine, Nursing, Pharmacy, Physical Therapy, Dietary and other identified disciplines, a plan of care for patients is outlined based upon critical pathways. Collaboration among all the disciplines, including the patient and family, continues throughout the patient's stay. Staff registered nurses participate and maintain the system of managed care on their designated units. In conjunction with the Case Managers, RNs identify variances to the care plan and focus on opportunities to improve care. To further enhance the delivery of care, Case Managers are available to assist in the management of patients with difficult problems, and will do so across the continuum of care.

A schematic interpretation of the organization of roles, relationships, and activities was created. Figure 6.1 depicts the essential components of the CMPM.

Step 4: Obtain Commitment of Key Participants at All Levels of the Organization

The CM working group was keenly aware that for the project to be implemented, they had to engender the support and commitment of the key participants. The CM working group began to work with both the nursing personnel and physicians on each of the pilot units.

The CM working group members held informational sessions with each of the pilot units. The first sessions with the nursing personnel dealt with information about the case management delivery system project, the clinical nurse specialist/case management role, and the role of the nursing staff, and the sessions with the physicians focused on how case management would provide their patients with a consistently higher level of care. Each of the informational sessions was followed by discussion sessions. Because both

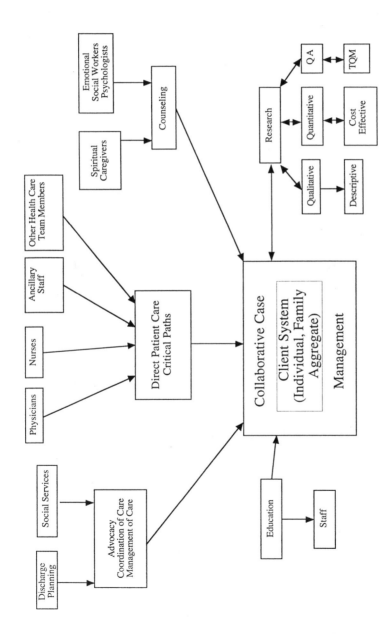

Figure 6.1. Case Management Practice Model (CMPM)

groups were given information regarding the CMPM project early in the development phase and were encouraged to discuss their feelings and concerns regarding the change to case management, both nursing personnel and physicians were supportive of the implementation and appeared to be committed to the project.

In addition to the informational sessions, all charge nurses were invited to an all-day workshop on case management. The workshop was led by an invited speaker, a clinical nurse specialist/case manager who had participated in the implementation of a case management system at a large urban medical center. Four of the CM working group members also presented a poster on the local CMPM implementation plans for the pilot units for which they were responsible.

Step 5: Identify Specific Measurable Objectives

Five objectives were developed to guide the project and to measure whether implementation had been successful:

1. Prepare clinical nurse specialists who will function as case managers on selected hospital units.
2. Develop critical paths for selected Diagnostic Related Groups (DRGs).
3. Facilitate multidisciplinary communication regarding patient care.
4. Coordinate the continuity of patient care through collaborative practice with physicians and auxiliary staff.
5. Evaluate the case management process and patient care outcomes on selected units.

Members of the CM working group developed specific program outlines and case management plans for the group of clients with whom they were currently working, based on information gathered at the interdisciplinary meetings, workshops, and programs. The following program outline resulted and was used in each of the targeted areas:

Phase 1
1. Educate staff on case management concepts and changes required for implementation.
2. Develop a system of variance review.
3. Develop a critical path template.
4. Meet with all physicians admitting patients to the unit to discuss the implementation of case management.
Phase 2
1. Develop critical paths for selected DRGs (e.g., cardiac, orthopedic, respiratory).

2. Continue staff/physician education.

3. Evaluate Phase 1 and revise plan as needed.

Phase 3

1. Begin case manager consultation for patients with complicated diagnoses (e.g., cardiac, orthopedic, respiratory).

2. Continue education for nursing and medical staff.

3. Evaluate Phase 2 and revise plan as needed.

Step 6: Establish Work Groups to Address the Objectives

The CM working group served as the primary work group, determining the timetable, strategies, activities, and resources necessary to facilitate implementation. One major resource identified was a computer system. The director of Computer Systems met with the CNS working group to discuss computer services necessary for the operation of the case management delivery system. After much discussion, it was decided that the system would be required to track length-of-stay and DRG variance. In addition, program capability would be needed to calculate cost-benefit analysis. The director of Computer Systems stated that the current mainframe PC system would be able to accommodate project needs. It was agreed that the evaluation data that measured patient, nurse, and physician satisfaction with the program implementation would be compiled and analyzed by the Center for Nursing Research at the University. The public relations director of the hospital was also contacted to assist the group in developing a list of proposed benefits for the constituencies that would be using the CMPM project. He also assisted the group in developing a series of strategies to facilitate implementation. The following are examples of the strategies that were implemented:

1. Marketing
   - Articles that discussed the need for and benefits of implementing a case management delivery system were written for both a regional hospital news magazine and an international newspaper.
   - Meetings were held with nurse managers and charge nurses discussing and clarifying case management and the implementation of the CMPM project.
   - Meetings were held with physician groups on each of the pilot units, at which critical paths were explained and case management implementation target dates were discussed.
2. Staff Education and Preparation
   - CM working group members were sent to a variety of conferences on case management.

- CM working group members met with the two groups mentioned above, as well as with the Dietary Department, Social Services Department, discharge planners, etc., to discuss each discipline's role in the implementation process.
- A case management workshop was planned and offered to the nurse manager and charge nurses.

Step 7: Use a Patient Care Focus to Involve Individuals From All Levels of the Organization

To involve all the hospital staff as well as market the case management delivery system, the CM working group developed a list of proposed benefits for each of the constituencies that would be involved in the CMPM project. The constituencies included patient/family, staff, physicians, ancillary staff (other than health care providers), hospital, and community (see Table 6.1).

Step 8: Build on Past Efforts to Avoid "Reinventing the Wheel"

During the initial stages of the project, hospital administration and the CM working group had agreed to maximize use of current resources and systems to curtail cost and maintain as much stability as possible within the system during the change process. An example of this was the computer system, as the existing system had a great deal of adaptability and application to the project. The CM working group and the Computer Systems Department were able to work cooperatively to utilize existing software to evaluate length of stay against DRGs. The software also permitted the inclusion of a section on nursing observations.

The faculty members of the group, however, were not as successful in finding instruments to measure patient, nurse, and physician satisfaction with the change to case management. Thus they developed three separate instruments to measure patient, nurse, and physician satisfaction. Further discussion of the development of the instruments is found in the evaluation section of this chapter.

Step 9: Educate Work Groups About the Interactive Planning Process

During the CMPM project development and implementation, the CM working group met regularly with all hospital personnel in the targeted areas. Group meetings, workshops, and in-service educational programs were offered. Each department within the hospital involved with the CMPM project participated in the programs. Although examples of interactive planning with the nurse managers and Computer Services Department personnel have been previously

TABLE 6.1 Proposed Constituency Benefits

1. Patient/Family
   a. Customized plan of care
   b. Continuity of care from admission to discharge
   c. Cost containment
   d. Improved patient outcome: e.g., decreased length of stay

2. Staff
   a. Increased patient/staff satisfaction
   b. Increased professionalism/enhanced clinical ladder
   c. Increased nurse/physician/departmental communication and relationships
   d. Increased accountability

3. Physician
   a. Improved patient outcomes
   b. Improved quality of care
   c. Improved compliance with Island Peer Review Organization (IPRO)/federal regulations
   d. Decreased frustration

4. Ancillary Staff
   a. Increased communication, teamwork, respect
   b. Enhanced holistic approach
   c. Proactive referrals of appropriate patients
   d. Anticipated care by each discipline

5. Hospital
   a. Mission fulfilled
   b. Increased patient/family/staff/physician satisfaction
   c. Decreased length of stay in relation to DRGs, cost reduction
   d. Increased quality, compliance with regulatory standards, IPRO

6. Community
   a. Resource for the community
   b. Provision of cost-effective care
   c. Provision of leadership for health care in the 21st century
   d. Identified community needs met

discussed, an example of the work with the orthopedic physicians developed when the CM working group met with them to explain the project and the proposed critical paths and care maps that the orthopedic CNS had developed. The orthopedic CNS had developed the drafts to determine if the physicians would approve the use of the critical paths and care maps for their patients. The orthopedic physicians were extremely enthusiastic about both the critical paths and care maps and wanted to know if they could be used at another area hospital where they admitted patients (see Table 6.2). All departments involved in the CMPM project were involved in similar interactive planning activities during the development and implementation of the project.

TABLE 6.2 The Orthopedic Care Management Plan

Goal: Length of stay will be decreased and delivery of quality care will be improved within effective and appropriate time frames. Case management will be implemented with selected orthopedic patients.

Phase 1
   Implement critical path for patients with total hip replacement on Unit 1 by March 1, 1993.

Phase 2
   Implement critical path for patients with total knee replacement on Unit 2 by May 1, 1993.

Phase 3
   Implement critical paths for patients with diagnosis of fractured hip, fractured distal femur, fractured fibula, and fractured tibia on Unit 2 by July 1, 1993.

Phase 4
   Implement case management for complicated orthopedic patients by August 1, 1993.

Step 10: Develop a Comprehensive, Ongoing Communication Plan

During implementation, which is still ongoing, strategies are being devised to communicate effectively with all departments that are involved in the CMPM project. Meetings, newsletters, in-service educational programs, and informal discussion groups are continuing. Evaluation research conducted as a result of the implementation will be shared with the staff to demonstrate whether the CMPM project is making a difference. At present, the case management practice model has been accepted and implemented by the hospital staff.

EVALUATION OF THE CASE MANAGEMENT PRACTICE MODEL

To evaluate the effectiveness of the CMPM of nursing care in this hospital, it was necessary to focus on both client- and system-centered variables.

Client-Centered Variables

Because one of the purposes of case management is to assist the patient and his or her family in the coordination of care throughout the hospitalization period and transition to either home or a long-term care facility, patient satisfaction with the case management approach had to be evaluated. A Patient Satisfaction Instrument was developed to measure this variable. The instrument was developed through a focus group approach, using the CM working group to generate dimensions related to the client.

Individual patient length of stay was also an important client-centered variable, as was the achievement of identified clinical and financial outcomes for the institution within a set time frame.

System-Centered Variables

Nursing staff satisfaction and physician satisfaction were identified as important components of the evaluation process. Length of stay and cost analysis were also included as system-centered variables.

An important component of any case management system is the computerization of data. Data are analyzed to measure changes in individual and unit service needs and to correlate client and system variables for effective use of resources. Integration of information from every department is necessary to analyze outcome and cost trends, and integrated patient information is also essential for the scheduling changes necessary to provide responsive staffing for patient and institutional needs. These data also allow comparative studies that examine outcomes between units or between hospitals.

Development of Evaluation Instruments

During CM working group meetings, the dimensions of the case management role were delineated. The dimensions used to develop the instruments for the patient, nursing staff, and physician groups can be found in Table 6.3.

Characteristics of each dimension were identified and used to guide the development of instrument items. A Likert-scale format with a 5-point scale was used. Respondents selected *strongly agree, agree, don't know, disagree,* or *strongly disagree* in response to the items. See Table 6.4 for sample items from the patient, nursing staff, and physician satisfaction instruments.

The evaluation of this case management project is under way at the present time and complete data are not yet available. Early indications show that patients and families feel their needs are being better met. Patients are positive about having one nurse identified as their manager. Staff outcomes include increased feelings of autonomy and control over patient care and improved job satisfaction. The continuity of care that includes participation in discharge planning has begun to give the nurses a greater sense of fulfillment. Physicians whose patients are on the pilot units appreciate the central coordination of care for their patients and the benefits offered by a multidisciplinary approach. The case management approach includes patient and family input into the planning of care and has begun to fully utilize existing resources while encouraging a multidisciplinary team approach.

TABLE 6.3 Dimensions of the Case Management Role

---

1. Dimensions of Case Management Applicable to Patients
   a. Participative care
   b. Multidisciplinary care
   c. Patient-focused care
   d. Aftercare
   e. Family involvement

2. Dimensions of Case Management Applicable to Nursing Staff
   a. Relationships with clinical nurse specialist and colleagues on the multidisciplinary team
   b. Job satisfaction and satisfaction with case management
   c. Opportunity for professional development—preparation to take on new role
   d. Ability to influence patient outcomes and delivery of care—ability to provide continuity of care
   e. Increased opportunity for autonomy and accountability

3. Dimensions of Case Management applicable to Physicians
   a. Obstacles to the delivery of care
   b. Collaboration and multidisciplinary team concept
   c. Aftercare and continuity
   d. Clinical competence of the staff delivering the care
   e. Patient outcomes

To be successful, the CMPM project must demonstrate that costs and length of stay can be reduced while the quality of care is maintained. The quality will be demonstrated through the attainment of specified goals on critical pathways for identified patient groups.

SUMMARY

The original goal of the CM working group was to develop a model of case management that would help increase the satisfaction of the clients and staff while still maintaining quality and cost-effective care. The CMPM, which developed during and as a result of the case management project, was based on a framework that outlined the objectives and roles of the CNS/case manager, physicians, and ancillary personnel involved in patient care.

The pilot study thus far indicates that collaboration is necessary within the various departments. Existing resources (e.g., computer systems and continuing education) should be utilized where appropriate to facilitate the implementation of a new practice model while keeping costs at a minimum. Cost savings are also anticipated as a result of the reconfiguration of the CNS/case manager role, as well as increased nursing staff satisfaction as their role is enhanced. Active involvement and acceptance from the nurses, physicians, and ancillary staff are essential for the project to succeed. It was found that discussing the

TABLE 6.4 Excerpts From the Satisfaction Instruments

---

1. Patient Satisfaction Instrument
   a. The nurse and the physician work closely together in caring for me during my illness.
   b. I feel very confident that the nurses are doing things that are in my best interest.
2. Nursing Staff Satisfaction Instrument
   a. My current job situation offers opportunities for me to practice autonomously.
   b. I feel confident in my ability to give high-level patient care.
3. Physician Satisfaction Instrument
   a. Collaboration and teamwork lead to improved patient outcomes.
   b. My patients are receiving excellent care from a multidisciplinary health care team.

---

project early and continuously during implementation was extremely helpful in increasing acceptance. As a result of the development of the critical paths and care maps, patient and family participation increased; this resulted in increased satisfaction and connections with the system of care. Involvement of all constituencies (physicians, case managers, staff nurses, ancillary staff, patients, and families) in the CMPM model helped to reduce redundancy and create a smooth transition between hospital and home or long-term care facility. Integration of the consultants into all components is necessary. This project would have been more quickly developed if they had been included in every meeting rather than once or twice monthly. The consultants would have also been able to test the instruments as each pilot unit instituted the case management model, rather than waiting to test until the project had been implemented. Finally, a single individual should be identified early as the case management project leader. This helps both in eliminating confusion about who is responsible for moving the project forward and in coordinating all constituencies. When the project leader was changed without the group's approval, the project was ultimately set back several months because trust had to be developed with the CM working group and the various constituencies involved in the project. However, results from the project thus far indicate success in reaching the original goal.

The instruments still require validation. Reliability will be ascertained as the instrument continues to be tested and sample size increases. The CMPM model also requires testing and validation to see if a smooth transition from hospital to home or a long-term care facility actually results from its use.

NOTE

1. Although it is a goal of the CMPM project to be implemented throughout the hospital, the definition here reflects only the pilot units.

REFERENCES

American Nurses Association. (1988). *Nursing case management.* Kansas City, MO: Author.

Bolton, L. B., Aydin, C., Popolow, G., & Ramseyer, J. (1992). Ten steps for managing organizational change. *Journal of Nursing Administration, 22*(6), 14-20.

Cronin, C. J., & Makleburst, J. (1989). Case-managed care: Capitalizing on the CNS. *Nursing Management, 20*(3), 38-39, 42-47.

Del Togno-Armanasco, V., Olivas, G., & Harter, A. S. (1989). Developing an integrated nursing case management model. *Nursing Management, 20*(10), 26-29.

Delahanty, P. M., Graves, R. A., & Hoffman, T. (1993). Case study: Managing care in a community hospital. In K. Kelly (Ed.), *Managing nursing care: Promises and pitfalls* (pp. 103-114). St. Louis: C. V. Mosby.

McKenzie, C., Torkelson, N., & Holt, M. (1989). Care and cost: Nursing case management improves both. *Nursing Management, 20*(10), 30-34.

Pittman, K. (1991, November/December). "Care": A case management model for empowering hospital nurses. *Florida Nurse, 4,* 6.

Schull, D. E., Tosch, P., & Wood, M. (1992). Clinical nurse specialists as collaborative care managers. *Nursing Management, 23*(3), 30-33.

Weinstein, R. (1991). Hospital case management: The path to empowering nurses. *Pediatric Nursing, 17,* 289-293.

Wyers, M. E. A., Grove, S. K., & Pastorino, C. (1986). Clinical nurse specialist: In search of the right role. *Nursing and Health Care, 4,* 203-207.

Zander, K. (1988). Managed care within acute care settings: Design and implementation via nursing case management. *Health Care Supervisor, 6*(2), 27-43.

Tracking and Analyzing Variances From CareMaps™

Colleen J. Goode　　*Almira T. Hinton*
Jean Barry Walker　*Roxanne Mills*
Vicki Ibarra　　　*Teresa Hamilton*
Greg Clancy　　　*Jan Reighard*

When critical paths or CareMaps are used in health care organizations as guidelines for providing care, tracking and analysis of variances from the Maps are essential activities that must be carried out by nurse case managers and members of the multidisciplinary team that develop the CareMap. Variance data provide the evaluation component for determining resource use and outcomes from use of a CareMap. Issues related to data collection, management, and analysis are discussed, and the necessity for goal setting and feedback is described.

Patient care is a complex process, resulting from the integration of the knowledge, skills, and actions of many professional health disciplines; the quality of the care a patient receives is an outcome of these combined efforts (Pike et al., 1993). Unfortunately, many of the activities to assess and improve the quality of this care are done by one discipline in isolation from the other involved disciplines. Identifying and solving quality problems in a vacuum have led to fragmentation of care, redundant and inadequate quality improvement

---

AUTHORS' NOTE: CareMap™ is a registered trademark of the Center for Case Management, South Natick, Massachusetts, and is used by permission.

programs, and, often, frustration for the members of the various disciplines. Because the provision of patient care is interdependent, it is reasonable that quality improvement and review efforts should also be multidisciplinary.

New systems of care that include multidisciplinary practice guidelines in the form of a critical path or CareMap with tracking and analysis of variances from the CareMap are being implemented in hospitals throughout the United States. These new care systems are a significant step toward integrated, multidisciplinary quality improvement programs. Research has shown that the use of a CareMap can decrease costs and improve patient outcomes (Blegen, Reiter, Goode, & Murphy, in press; Cohen, 1991; Goode, 1993; Ogilvie-Harris, Botsford, & Hawker, 1993). The CareMap eliminates nonessential care and sequences the care provided by physicians, nurses, and other key providers throughout an episode of care. It decreases the variation in practice, improves efficiency, reduces costs, and improves quality. Experience has shown that a multidisciplinary approach to developing the CareMap is essential for success (American Health Consultants, 1993; Goode & Blegen, 1993a). All disciplines that provide care to the patient population for which the CareMap is being developed should contribute to the content of the clinical guideline and to the tracking and analysis of variance from the guideline.

This chapter addresses the process of variance tracking; issues related to the collection, management, and analysis of data; and the necessity of a feedback loop for continuous outcomes evaluation and management.

DEFINING VARIANCE TRACKING AND ANALYSIS

Variance tracking and variance analysis are methodologies for measuring resource use and outcomes when a CareMap is used. When deviations from the CareMap occur and patients and clinicians who provide care do not follow the CareMap as outlined, these deviations are recorded as variances. The CareMap defines the process components of care, and the variance tracking and analysis are the evaluation components of the care. A variance tracking form is used by clinicians to record key activities and outcomes that do not occur or occur earlier than outlined on the CareMap. Variances are recorded by clinicians from all disciplines as they occur. Variance data are collated and aggregated for specific patient populations and fed back to the multidisciplinary team for analysis.

PROCESS OF VARIANCE TRACKING

Establishment of a system in which all providers from all disciplines record variances from the CareMap is a challenging undertaking. It requires ongoing

education and innovation to find ways so that clinicians do not have to duplicate entries on the patient chart. The University of Iowa Hospitals and Clinics (UIHC) began with a variance tracking record that was modeled after the one used at Toronto General Hospital and is displayed in Figure 7.1. After using this tool for about a year, the clinicians were able to identify multiple problems with its use in the clinical setting. First, the form took too long to complete. Second, clinicians were not properly coding reasons for the variance because the categories were not mutually exclusive and inter-rater reliability was lacking. Third, the quantity of variance information was overwhelming, and often variances did not seem to have significant impact on the outcomes. For all these reasons, a new multidisciplinary variance tracking form was designed and is displayed in Figure 7.2. The variance tracking record and the CareMap are a permanent part of the patient record at UIHC.

The goal was to develop a new tracking record that would be valid, reliable, and user friendly for the clinician. A hospital committee of case managers representing several patient populations determined that only variances from the key intermediate goals, key critical path activities, and all final outcomes would be tracked. Each multidisciplinary team would identify the key events most critical to achievement of outcomes. Through this method, content validity of the tool would be established by the clinical experts on each multidisciplinary CareMap development team. Classification of the variances as systems, provider, or patient problems would be done by the nurse case managers assigned to the specific patient population. Inter-rater reliability could then be established for the case managers. This enhanced coding because it was impossible to establish reliability among multiple clinicians who were coding information as they recorded it on the tracking record.

Each CareMap is accompanied by a set of preprinted physician orders. The nurse case manager and the physician add and delete from these orders to meet the needs of individual patients. For example, medications may be changed due to patient drug allergies, or additional medications and treatments may be ordered because the patient has diabetes. Changes made to the preprinted orders and CareMap on initial assessment or on admission are not recorded as variances. However, physician and nurse orders added after this time are recorded and become a part of the variance tracking data.

At UIHC, key intermediate goals and key critical path activities are called *key events*. When new CareMaps are developed for a specific patient population, the multidisciplinary team that develops the CareMap hypothesizes which key events will have an effect on length of stay, costs, and/or patient satisfaction. As Figures 7.1. and 7.2 demonstrate, shading has been added on the CareMap record to highlight key events. This helps staff to identify the key activities and

A-21

CAREMAP TRACKING RECORD

DATE

HOSP. NO.

NAME

BIRTH DATE

ADDRESS

Appendix A

File most recent sheet of this number ON BOTTOM.

IF NOT IMPRINTED, PLEASE PRINT HOSP.NO., NAME AND LOCATION.

A 21

CareMap Name and Number _____ UIHC Expected LOS _____

Date of Surgery _____   Discharge Date _____   Discharge Unit _____

Hosp Days to Date	Actual Care-Map Day	CAREMAP Problem No. (see CareMap)	Critical Path No. (select 1 to 9)	VARIANCE/COMMENTS	SOURCE Goal/Event Occurr. (select 1 to 4)	Cate-gory (select A to D)	Reason (select 1 to 16)	VARIANCE ACTIONS	Date, Name, and Position

PROBLEM NO.	CRITICAL PATH NO.	GOAL/EVENT OCCURRENCE	CATEGORY	REASON	
0 Problem not on CareMap 1, 2, 3 ... as on CareMap	1 Consults 2 Tests 3 Treatments 4 Medications 5 Diet 6 Activity 7 Teaching 8 Discharge 9 All events for CareMap Day not met	1 Did not occur 2 Early 3 Late 4 Additional	A Patient/Family B Clinician/Caregiver C System/Institutions D Community	1 Patient condition 2 Pt/Family decision 3 Pt/Family availability 4 Pt/Family other 5 Physician order 6 Caregiver decision 7 Caregiver response time 8 Caregiver other	9 Bed availability 10 Information/Data avail. 11 Supplies/Equip. avail. 12 Department closed 13 Hospital other 14 Placement/Home care availability 15 Transportation avail. 16 Community other

CareMap™ is a registered trademark of The Center for Case Management, South Natick, MA. and is used by permission.

NID013 6/92   THE UNIVERSITY OF IOWA HOSPITALS AND CLINICS

(side tabs: B CLIN. NOTES, C LABORATORY, D X-RAY EXAM, E CONSULTATION, F SPEC. EXAM, G THERAPY, H PATHOLOGY, I DIAGNOSIS)

Figure 7.1. Variance Tracking Record and CareMap Formerly Used at UIHC

goals and serves as a reminder to the practitioners to document variances related to these activities and goals. Also, preprinting key events on the variance tracking record assists caregivers in the documentation of variation that occurs. After the CareMap has been implemented for some time and data collection

A-21		DATE	
CAREMAP TRACKING RECORD		HOSP. NO.	Appendix B
		NAME	
		BIRTHDATE	
		ADDRESS	
• File most recent sheet of this number ON BOTTOM •		IF NOT IMPRINTED, PLEASE PRINT DATE, HOSP. NO., NAME AND LOCATION	

CareMap Name _____   CareMap ID# _____

CareMap Day/Sequence Date/Initials	Key Event	Variance/Reason	Action

INITIALS/SIGNATURES

_____ / _____   _____ / _____   _____ / _____

_____ / _____   _____ / _____   _____ / _____

_____ / _____   _____ / _____   _____ / _____

CareMap™ is a registered trademark of the Center for Case Management, South Natick, MA and is used by permission.
The University of Iowa Hospitals and Clinics

1/10/95

Figure 7.2. Variance Tracking Record and CareMap Currently Used at UIHC

has identified barriers that have delayed patient progress along the CareMap, the multidisciplinary team revises and makes additions and deletions from the key event list for that CareMap. For example, a key event defined for the Percutaneous Transluminal Coronary Angioplasty (PTCA) CareMap was removal of the femoral sheath. After using the CareMap for a few months and analyzing the data that were recorded, the team determined that they could make the data more meaningful by identifying the reasons for delays in removal of the femoral sheath, such as dissection, elevated bleeding time, or late arrival to the unit. These specific reasons for possible delay have now been added to the variance tracking record.

Examples of key events for the CareMap developed for mothers having a cesarean birth include pain control rating at a level that is not acceptable by the patient, IV not discontinued within 36 hours postoperatively, prophylactic antibiotics in excess of a one-time dose for mothers with premature rupture of the membranes, and hemoglobin and hematocrit less than or equal to 8% and 24%, respectively. These key events were established after analysis of several months' variance data.

VARIANCE ANALYSIS

It is essential that both concurrent analysis by the clinicians and analysis of aggregate data by the multidisciplinary team be part of the system of analysis. Concurrent analysis provides the opportunity to take action immediately to bring the patient into compliance with expected outcomes. An example of the need for concurrent analysis is evident in data from the cesarean section CareMap. If a patient rates her pain greater than a 3 on a 0 to 10 scale and states that this pain level is not tolerable, a variance is recorded and action is taken immediately to provide pain relief.

Retrospective analysis of the data obtained from review of variation derived from the use of the CareMap for groups of patients provides a means to identify variance trends for specific patient populations. For example, analysis by the multidisciplinary team of aggregate data for patients who were having a cesarean birth indicated that there were delays in discharge because prescriptions were not being written and filled in a timely manner. A plan was enacted whereby prescriptions were stamped by the unit clerk with the patient's name and placed on the chart for rounds on the day before dismissal. These prescriptions were sent to the pharmacy and returned to the unit the evening before discharge. Aggregate data also indicated that the number of patients rating their pain above a 3 (0-10 scale) was excessive. A new pain management plan was implemented whereby oral meds were started earlier and additional pain medications were added to the Map to supplement either the epidural or the PCA pump medications. This resulted in improved pain management and a significant reduction in variation.

At UIHC, variance data have been used to indicate where additional staff training is needed, to modify the CareMap, and to identify needed systems changes. For example, some physicians were ordering more dosages of antibiotics than the CareMap specified for mothers who had premature rupture of the membranes. Additional physician staff education was needed. Physicians on the multidisciplinary team gathered studies related to antibiotic treatment of premature rupture and distributed and discussed these with the residents and faculty physicians. Education of the physicians had a significant impact on decreasing variances in this area.

A systems problem was identified when data revealed variances due to teaching delays for patients who did not speak English. This was particularly a problem on weekends. The Social Services Department adjusted staffing to provide better coverage on weekends, and additional written information and videos in Spanish were also produced. Variances related to teaching delays for non-English speaking mothers were eliminated.

Aggregate analysis identified the need for CareMap changes for the PTCA patient population. The multidisciplinary team determined that a number of patients were outliers because they were not going home within the length of stay outlined on the CareMap. Aggregate data indicated that the PTCA Care-Map worked well for those patients with stable angina and for whom the PTCA was successful in opening the blocked coronary artery. However, when the CareMap was used for patients who had a PTCA to revascularize heart tissue post MI, patients required extended hospitalization. The team decided to place PTCA CareMap patients who had had an MI on the post-MI CareMap 24 hours after the PTCA procedure until they completed their rehabilitation. Thus patients with stable angina would have the standard PTCA CareMap and be discharged within 24 hours. The post-MI patients who had had a PTCA would go on the MI CareMap after 24 hours on the standard PTCA CareMap. The goal of differentiating the PTCA population into subgroups and planning appropriate activities for the patient groups was a direct outcome of aggregate data analysis. Now that these PTCA subgroups are differentiated, further information can be collected and CareMaps adjusted for each group.

Data Management

Case Managers enter data into a relational database (Paradox), and data are then displayed in reports. Descriptive statistics, such as frequency counts, ranges, and percentages, are used to display and summarize the data. If the sample size is large enough, a mean also can be calculated. By having the data in a relational database, it is possible to connect key events to outcomes. For example, for all patients who exceed the optimal prescribed length of stay, the key events not met can be determined. Data are then displayed in bar graphs, line graphs, and other visual forms.

The current paper-based system for collecting, analyzing, and displaying data is very labor intensive. Early on, we learned that collecting unlimited amounts of data was overwhelming and did not contribute to improved outcomes. Streamlining and focusing only on collection of essential data has helped tremendously. Even then, it is readily evident to clinicians from all disciplines that the variance tracking system must be automated. We currently have a team working on automating this process. The team is cochaired by a physician and a nurse. An automated system that tracks variances and collates and trends them over time will enhance accuracy of the data and improve the efficiency of the nurse case managers. They can then be freed up to do more care managing to keep patients on track on the CareMap.

FEEDBACK AND GOAL SETTING
FOR CONTINUOUS QUALITY IMPROVEMENT

Collection and analysis of the statistical data from CareMaps is a strong component of the outcomes management program at UIHC. The clinical data from the CareMap are combined with financial data, measures of patient satisfaction, and measures of functional status to provide information for outcomes evaluation and management.

Office of Outcomes Evaluation and Management

Development of multidisciplinary practice guidelines is really a quality management process. When CareMaps are developed, they address "doing the right thing," or efficiency and appropriateness. Through variance analysis, it is determined whether the "right things are done well." The "right things done well" include availability, timeliness, and effectiveness of tests, procedures, treatments, and services, as well as continuity and efficiency of services. In essence, through variance documentation and analysis, a database is developed for quality improvement.

This database is essential to the personnel in the UIHC Office of Outcomes Evaluation and Management. The purpose of this office, established in 1994, is to improve the quality and value of services provided to customers. This is accomplished through assessment, analysis, and improvement of clinical outcomes and operational efficiency. Analysis of variance data is part of the mission of the Office of Outcomes Evaluation and Management. Variance data identify system and clinical processes in need of further analysis. Outcomes data verify the effectiveness of clinical processes as well as the need for modifications in these processes. The case management/project manager in the Office of Outcomes Evaluation and Management assists with the formulation, implementation, and use of databases for clinical and administrative decision making. Use of variance data by the Office of Outcomes Evaluation and Management facilitates comparison of sets of data over time. Summary data can be provided to customers for use in informed decision making.

Feedback and Goal Setting

Variance tracking integrated with an interdisciplinary feedback and goal-setting mechanism provides the foundation for an ongoing program of continuous quality improvement. Goal setting has received a wide array of empirical support for its positive effect on individual and team performance (Latham & Yukl, 1975; Locke, 1978; Locke & Latham, 1990; Locke, Frederick, Lee, & Bobko, 1984). The results are consistent: Goal setting enhances performance. Goals that are specific rather than broad, self-set rather than imposed, and challenging but achievable are the most effective in motivating individuals (Manz, 1992; Manz & Sims, 1989). In addition, a review of 100 experimental studies indicated that feedback, when coupled with goal setting, promoted even higher levels of performance (Locke, Shaw, & Saari, 1981). Stull (1986), in a study of nurse goal setting and performance feedback, found enhanced staff nurse performance when both goal setting and feedback were used. Numerous other authors have concurred that objective feedback is a potent method to enhance performance, motivation, and job satisfaction (Brannon & Bucher, 1989; Roedal & Nystrom, 1988; Seybolt, 1986).

Variance data are of no use if they are not shared with the multidisciplinary team and with the clinicians who provide the care. The goal is to reduce unnecessary variance that may increase costs or decrease quality. The most difficult part of the process may be to change behaviors of clinicians. The way clinicians of all disciplines carry out their work is deeply embedded in the culture of the organization and/or is a reflection of their training. However, clinicians' commitment to provide the highest quality care possible for their patients and the regular feedback of relevant and focused quality data can be potent motivators for the acceptance of the need for a change in practice (Argyris, 1970; Goode & Blegen, 1993b). Professional commitment, a well-developed feedback mechanism coupled with the identification of needed practice changes, and the implementation of an ongoing multidisciplinary goal-setting process to achieve these changes provide the foundation for a multidisciplinary program of clinical excellence and continuous quality improvement.

This model is essential if we are to survive against a background of steadily increasing cost and diminishing operational margins. Through variance analysis, we can obtain quantitative information from which we can learn and take action to improve the processes of care. In the typical hospital environment, much of the clinical and financial data has not been shared. Through variance analysis, these feedback data are given directly to the clinicians who control resource use.

CONCLUSION

The CareMap and variance tracking form are tools used by all disciplines to guide practice and to evaluate and manage the processes and outcomes of care. The contribution of CareMaps and variance tracking and analysis to ensuring the financial integrity of the hospital is widely recognized in today's health care environment. Restructuring is going on in most health care organizations, and reengineering of the clinical processes of care by use of CareMaps and variance analysis is common. This care management system is an important investment in continuous quality improvement at the bedside (Zander, 1993). The variance tracking system will provide relevant concurrent and aggregate data for continuous improvement of care. However, fundamental to an ongoing program of continuous quality improvement is an innovative, clinically knowledgeable, collaborative multidisciplinary team made up of members with an innate desire to provide care that is reflective of "best practice."

REFERENCES

American Health Consultants. (1993). Why Alliant and Toronto Hospitals are reassessing hundreds of paths. *Hospital Case Management, 1*(3), 41-45.

Argyris, C. (1970). *Intervention theory and method.* Reading, MA: Addison-Wesley.

Blegen, M. A., Reiter, R., Goode, C. J., & Murphy, R. (in press). Outcomes of hospital-based managed care: Cost and quality. *Journal of Obstetrics and Gynecology.*

Brannon, D., & Bucher, J. (1989). Quality assurance feedback as a nursing management strategy. *Hospital and Health Services Administration, 34,* 547-558.

Cohen, E. L. (1991). Nursing case management: Does it pay? *Journal of Nursing Administration, 21*(4), 20-25.

Goode, C. J. (1993). *Evaluation of patient and staff outcomes with hospital-based managed care.* Unpublished doctoral dissertation, University of Iowa.

Goode, C. J., & Blegen, M. A. (1993a). Developing a CareMap for patients with a cesarean birth: A multidisciplinary process. *Journal of Perinatal and Neonatal Nursing, 7*(2), 40-49.

Goode, C. J., & Blegen, M. A. (1993b). Development and evaluation of a research-based management intervention. *Journal of Nursing Administration, 23*(4), 61-66.

Latham, G. P., & Yukl, G. A. S. (1975). A review of research on the application of goal-setting in organizations. *Academy of Management Journal, 18,* 824-845.

Locke, E. A. (1978). The ubiquity of goal-setting in theories and approaches to employee motivation. *Academy of Management Review, 3,* 594-601.

Locke, E., Frederick, E., Lee, C., & Bobko, P. (1984). Effect of self-efficacy, goals, and task strategies of task performance. *Journal of Applied Psychology, 69,* 241-251.

Locke, E., & Latham, G. P. (1990). *A theory of goal setting and task performance.* Englewood Cliffs, NJ: Prentice Hall.

Locke, E. A., Shaw, K. N., & Saari, L. M. (1981). Goal-setting and task performance: 1969-1980. *Psychological Bulletin, 90,* 125-152.

Manz, C. (1992). *Mastering self-leadership: Empowering yourself for personal excellence.* Englewood Cliffs, NJ: Prentice Hall.

Manz, C., & Sims, H. P. (1989). *Superleadership.* New York: Berkley.

Ogilvie-Harris, D., Botsford, D., & Hawker, R. (1993). Elderly patients with hip fractures: Improved outcomes with the use of care maps with high-quality medical and nursing protocols. *Journal of Orthopaedic Trauma, 7,* 428-437.

Pike, A., McHugh, M., Canney, K. C., Miller, N. E., Reiley, P., & Seibert, C. P. (1993). A new architecture for quality assurance: Nurse-physician collaboration. *Journal of Nursing Care Quality, 7*(3), 1-8.

Roedal, R., & Nystrom, P. (1988). Nursing jobs and satisfaction. *Nursing Management, 19*(2), 34-38.

Seybolt, J. W. (1986). Dealing with premature turnover. *Journal of Nursing Administration, 16,* 26-32.

Stull, M. K. (1986). Staff nurse performance: Effects of goal-setting and performance feedback. *Journal of Nursing Administration, 16*(7/8), 26-30.

Zander, K. (1993). Quantifying, managing and improving quality, Part IV: The retrospective use of variance. *New Definition, 8*(1), 1-3.

CHAPTER 8

Successful Strategies for Implementing AHCPR Clinical Practice Guidelines

Victoria M. Steelman

This chapter describes the process of implementing clinical practice guidelines in a large, tertiary teaching hospital. Barriers to utilizing research in practice are reviewed along with responsibilities of nurse administrators. The Iowa Model of Research-Based Practice to Promote Quality Care is presented as a conceptual framework for implementation of clinical practice guidelines. Key strategies for implementation and for measuring the impact on patient, staff, and fiscal outcomes are presented.

Nurse administrators are experiencing increasing demands from accrediting agencies, third-party payers, and patients to demonstrate that care provided is appropriate, timely, and cost-effective. One strategy proposed to meet these demands is implementation of clinical practice guidelines. The Agency for Health Care Policy and Research (AHCPR) has taken a leading role in developing clinical practice guidelines at the national level. Written by panels of experts, including nurses, these guidelines synthesize the knowledge of specific patient problems and outline a range of multidisciplinary treatment options from which the clinician may select. To date, the AHCPR has published 10 guidelines, and others are under development.[1]

AUTHOR'S NOTE: I acknowledge Colleen Goode, PhD, RN, Associate Director, University of Iowa Hospitals and Clinics and Interim Director of Nursing, for her leadership in research utilization, and the nursing staff throughout the department who have been instrumental in implementing clinical practice guidelines at UIHC.

TABLE 8.1 Barriers Related to the Research and Presentation

---

1. Statistical analysis is not understandable.

2. The relevant literature is not compiled in one place.

3. Implications for practice are not made clear.

4. Research reports/articles are not readily available.

5. The research has not been replicated.

6. The research is not reported clearly and at audience level of understanding.

7. The research is not relevant to the nurse's practice.

8. The nurse is uncertain whether to believe the results of the research.

9. The literature reports conflicting results.

10. The research has methodological inadequacies.

11. Research reports/articles are not published fast enough.

12. The conclusions drawn from the research are not justified.

SOURCE: Funk et al. (1991).

By compiling the relevant literature in one place and synthesizing it into an easily understood form, the authors of the guidelines minimize many barriers to using research in clinical practice. Barriers related to the research itself and its presentation have been identified by clinicians as leading reasons for not implementing research findings (Funk, Champagne, Wiess, & Tournquist, 1991; see Table 8.1). Clinicians are confused by conflicting results and statistical analyses that are not easily understood. The panels of experts authoring the guidelines have evaluated the scientific merit of the research, reported it clearly and concisely, and clearly identified implications for practice. Although barriers related to the research and its presentation have been addressed, other barriers also hinder clinicians, particularly those related to the setting and the nurse. Lack of authority and time have been identified by clinicians as the leading reasons for not utilizing research, and 8 of the top 10 barriers identified relate to the setting itself (see Table 8.2). The support needed from administrators and physicians is often seen as lacking. These barriers, similar to those identified in other studies, are often overlooked or underestimated (Champion & Leach, 1989; Miller & Messenger, 1978; Pettengill, Gillies, & Clark, 1994).

SETTING THE STAGE FOR SUCCESS

The nurse administrator is in a key position to ensure the successful implementation of clinical practice guidelines by first minimizing barriers related to the setting (Goode & Bulechek, 1992). However, because of the multidisciplinary nature of the guidelines, implementation poses a significant challenge,

TABLE 8.2 Barriers Related to the Setting

1. The nurse does not feel that he or she has enough authority to change patient care procedures.
2. There is insufficient time on the job to implement new ideas.
3. Physicians will not cooperate with implementation.
4. Administrators will not allow implementation.
5. Other staff are not supportive of implementation.
6. The nurse feels that results are not generalizable to his or her own setting.
7. The facilities are inadequate for implementation.
8. The nurse does not have time to read research.

SOURCE: Funk et al. (1991).

particularly in a large teaching hospital. For example, nurses can affect the frequency and type of pain assessment and documentation but have little control over the type and amount of analgesics prescribed. To address this challenge, the Department of Nursing of the University of Iowa Hospitals and Clinics (UIHC) has developed a successful program to implement clinical practice guidelines. It begins with a strong organizational commitment to a research-based practice (Goode & Bulechek, 1992).

Addressing organizational barriers to utilizing research throughout the nursing department has set the stage for a successful program. The director of nursing at UIHC, nationally renowned for research utilization, encourages it both verbally and by demonstration. The value of research is in the mission statement of the hospital and the philosophy and objectives of the department of nursing. Both research conduct and utilization have been incorporated into the strategic plan of the department. Each nursing division has a research committee that has been given the authority and responsibility to implement research in practice. The expectation to utilize research findings is in job descriptions and performance appraisals. The time spent implementing guidelines is supported throughout the department as an investment in improving the quality of patient care. For example, a committee working on implementation of the pain guidelines met for months to coordinate implementation. Supplies were provided for poster displays, and contributions of teams and individuals have been recognized in promotional brochures.

THE IOWA MODEL

To guide staff in decision making based on research, the Nursing Research Committee developed a conceptual model that is used for all research utiliza-

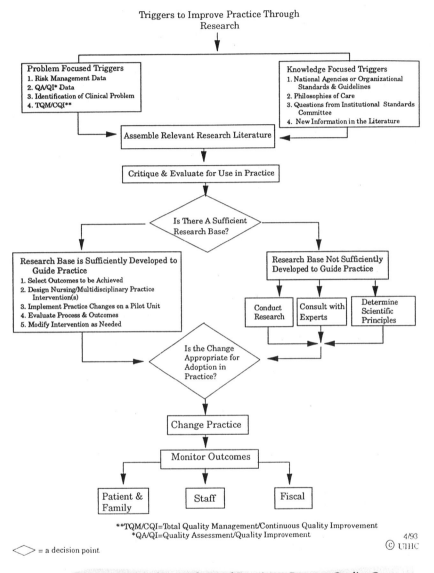

Figure 8.1. The Iowa Model of Research-Based Practice to Promote Quality Care

SOURCE: Dept. of Nursing of the University of Iowa Hospitals and Clinics. Reprinted with permission.

tion projects. The Iowa model for of research-based practice to promote quality care serves as a valuable tool for the process of implementing clinical practice guidelines (Titler et al., 1994; see Figure 8.1). In addition to being a conceptual framework, the model provides step-by-step direction to nurses, providing them with the autonomy to make research-based change while ensuring that key steps are not overlooked.

In the Iowa model, clinical practice guidelines serve as knowledge-focused triggers to improve the quality of patient care. The panel of experts authoring the guideline has done much of the initial work required for a research utilization project. The panel has assembled relevant research literature and critiqued and evaluated it for use in practice. Some of the interventions recommended in the guidelines are based on a research base sufficiently developed to guide practice. When the research base is not sufficiently developed to guide practice, the panel authoring the guideline provides expert opinion and makes recommendations on the range of acceptable treatment options available to the clinician. However, this work by the panel eliminates some of the group process needed to develop a commitment to a change. Therefore it is advisable to review the guidelines, one or two key research studies or meta-analyses published in the area, and any research on the topic published after the guideline was printed.

Once this has been completed, a committee determines if a change is appropriate for adoption in practice. This requires careful examination of several factors: the setting, the patient population, and current practice. This step is essential and must not be overlooked. For example, *Cataract in Adults: Management of Functional Impairment* (Cataract Management Guideline Panel, 1993) will have little application in a pediatric hospital, and *Sickle Cell Disease: Screening, Diagnosis, Management, and Counseling in Newborns and Infants* (Sickle Cell Disease Guideline Panel, 1993) will not apply to adult populations or patients of northern European descent. Guidelines may apply only to certain groups treated within an institution. At UIHC, the *Benign Prostatic Hyperplasia: Diagnosis and Treatment* guideline (Benign Prostatic Hyperplasia Guideline Panel, 1994) affects only one nursing division and one group of patients. Therefore a change could be limited to that division. Conversely, *Acute Pain Management: Operative or Medical Procedures and Trauma* (Acute Pain Management Guideline Panel, 1992a) applies to most nursing divisions and many patient populations. Therefore the focus of changes was much broader. Finally, the guideline is compared to current practice. At UIHC, staff were already compliant with some of the guidelines, such as *Cataract in Adults: Management of Functional Impairment* (Cataract Management Guideline Panel, 1993) and *Depression in Primary Care: Vol. 1. Detection and Diagnosis* (Depression Guideline Panel, 1993). However, when current standards and actual practice were compared with *Acute Pain Management: Operative or*

Medical Procedures and Trauma (Acute Pain Management Guideline Panel, 1992a) and *Pressure Ulcers in Adults: Prediction and Prevention* (Panel for the Prediction and Prevention of Pressure Ulcers in Adults, 1992), opportunities for improvement were identified.

CHANGE

Once it is determined that a change is desirable, alternatives are examined, and the best strategy is selected. The strategy selected depends on the level of multidisciplinary work required and the number of nursing units involved. For example, urology nurses found that changes needed for *Urinary Incontinence in Adults* (Urinary Incontinence Guideline Panel, 1992) were much less extensive than the changes recommended in *Acute Pain Management: Operative or Medical Procedures and Trauma* (Acute Pain Management Guideline Panel, 1992a). Approaches used at UIHC include (a) integration into care maps, (b) inclusion in new services, (c) incorporation into computerized protocols and standards, (d) patient education, (e) staff education, and (f) resource development.

Integration Into Care Maps

During the past 3 years, UIHC has implemented a case management program for various patient populations. Multidisciplinary teams have been established to standardize patient care through development of care maps identifying the usual needs and expected outcomes of specific groups of patients. Development of care maps provides an ideal mechanism for integration of guidelines, particularly those requiring multidisciplinary changes. The group process is already in place, and the team is accustomed to making decisions about patient care by consensus. For example, use of a standardized scale for pain assessment has been incorporated into care maps for surgical and C-section patients (Acute Pain Management Guideline Panel, 1992a). Treatments on these care maps include opioids for the immediate incisional pain, administered via epidural catheter or patient-controlled analgesia pump. On Day 2 of the map, the patient has progressed to oral analgesics and nonsteroidals (Acute Pain Management Guideline Panel, 1992a). Although current practice was consistent with *Cataract in Adults: Management of Functional Impairment* (Cataract Management Guideline Panel, 1993), this guideline was used as a basis for developing a care map for cataract patients. Patient education and follow-up appointments the day after surgery were included, as indicated in the guideline (Cataract Management Guideline Panel, 1993).

Inclusion in New Services

The guidelines are also reviewed when initiating new services. For example, when a new clinical cancer center was opened in 1993, a multidisciplinary committee was established to identify the services needed for this patient population. Consistent with *Management of Cancer Pain* (Management of Cancer Pain Guideline Panel, 1994), the committee incorporated a comprehensive pain history into patient care. A plan was implemented to provide multidisciplinary physical and cognitive-behavioral interventions as well as the pharmacological treatments. Because this committee is accustomed to making decisions as a team, implementation of the guidelines has been facilitated. The clinical nurse specialist (CNS) hired for the cancer center has expertise in cancer pain management and served as a reviewer for *Management of Cancer Pain* (Management of Cancer Pain Guideline Panel, 1994) prior to publication. This expertise has provided support for implementation of the guideline as well as a consultant for the staff for cancer pain issues.

Incorporation Into Computerized Protocols and Standards

For patients not on a care map, computerized nursing protocols and standards have been developed incorporating the guidelines into patient care. Acute pain and cancer pain protocols have been developed for adults, addressing frequency and type of assessments and pharmacological as well as nonpharmacological treatments. Similarly, a standard of care for pain management has been written for pediatric patients, including the use of pediatric pain scales advocated in *Acute Pain Management in Infants, Children, and Adolescents: Operative or Medical Procedures* (Acute Pain Management Guideline Panel, 1992b; Schmidt, Holida, Kleiber, Peterson, & Phearman, 1994). This endeavor has been very successful, resulting in many requests from other hospitals for copies. Using protocols has also been a successful strategy when guidelines do not require a multidisciplinary focus. For example, *Pressure Ulcers in Adults: Prediction and Prevention* (Panel for the Prediction and Prevention of Pressure Ulcers in Adults, 1992) outlined a number of independent nursing interventions. A pressure ulcer prevention protocol was developed that addresses desirable outcomes, use of the Braden Scale for systematic assessment of risk (Braden, 1989), interventions, and evaluation of these interventions as recommended in the guideline. *Urinary Incontinence in Adults* (Urinary Incontinence Guideline Panel, 1992) has also been implemented through a computerized protocol. This protocol includes assessment of urinary patterns and interventions such as behavioral techniques, catheterization, and patient education outlined in the guideline (Urinary Incontinence Guideline Panel, 1992). Because these protocols are on line, they can be accessed by nurses planning care for patients on any nursing unit throughout the hospital.

Patient Education

Clinical practice guidelines also address the need for patient and family education. Each guideline comes with a separate patient education brochure. These brochures were reviewed for relevance to the patient populations at UIHC and used as a reference when developing institution-specific patient education materials. Pediatric nurses developed two informational publications, *Helping Your Child With Pain Control* and *Use of PCA With the Pediatric Patient* (Schmidt et al., 1994). They are currently developing a third brochure about pain management in infants. Hospital-wide patient educational materials have also been developed for acute and cancer pain management in adults. Preoperative education includes frequency of pain assessment and use of scales. Patients are allowed to select a scale from a set of reliable tools available. They are also taught how to use a PCA pump and relaxation techniques.

Staff Education

Staff education has been an essential strategy to ensure the success of implementation of clinical practice guidelines. To determine what content was appropriate, nursing staff members were surveyed about their knowledge of the AHCPR guidelines. Responses demonstrated a minimal level of understanding of the guidelines. Therefore a comprehensive educational program was developed that is being presented to all nursing staff. The content of the program includes (a) the purpose of guidelines, (b) development process, (c) guidelines currently available, and (d) implementation of guidelines (Kraus, Fink, Hradek, & Sueppel, 1994).

Staff education has involved a number of centralized and unit-based activities to present content from different clinical practice guidelines. At the department level, *Pressure Ulcers in Adults: Prediction and Prevention* (Panel for the Prediction and Prevention of Pressure Ulcers in Adults, 1992) has been used for development of a continuing education program. A mandatory pain management course is being developed. Other programs have been decentralized. Critical care nurses have presented in-services on pressure ulcer prevention, and EENT nurses have presented in-services on pain management. Pediatric nurses have surveyed staff to determine the knowledge of nurses about pain management and have based educational programs on the results. Innovative posters have been developed to educate staff, information has been included in a divisional newsletter, and in-services have been provided (Schmidt et al., 1994). Resource notebooks on pain management have been made for each nursing unit. Orientation to Neurology, Surgery, and the Clinical Cancer Center has been modified to include content on pain management and pressure ulcer prevention. Other staff education activities have been undertaken in every nursing division.

Not all of the guidelines have required a change in clinical practice. When this has been the case, recognition is provided to the staff about the quality patient care being provided. For example, *Depression in Primary Care: Vol. 1. Detection and Diagnosis* (Depression Guideline Panel, 1993) was reviewed by the Psychiatric Nursing Division. The contents of the guideline (e.g., risk factors, symptoms, diagnosis, treatment plan, evaluation) were presented during grand rounds, and the information was circulated to all applicable nursing units. Because the care provided was already consistent with the guideline, staff were recognized for the high-level quality care they were providing.

Resource Development

In addition to staff education, changes in documentation have encouraged compliance, making standardized scales easily accessible and ensuring that staff have the resources they need to use the knowledge. We have incorporated changes into care maps, assessment forms, and flow sheets. For example, the admission assessment form for adults includes the Braden Scale to identify the level of risk for skin breakdown (Braden, 1989). Because the scale is on the form, nurses automatically complete the assessment. A pain history form has been developed for cancer pain and is routinely placed in the chart for oncology patients. In this manner, the form triggers questions that nurses need to ask when completing a baseline pain assessment. Flow sheets were developed to document pain, encouraging the use of standardized scales. To facilitate these assessments further, the scales were laminated and put on a ring at each patient's bedside. Pain resource manuals have been developed for each nursing unit to guide nurses in using appropriate interventions. These measures, in addition to staff education, have addressed the barriers to research utilization associated with the nurse (see Table 8.2; Funk et al., 1991).

MEASURING THE IMPACT

The last step of the Iowa model (Titler et al., 1994) is evaluation of staff, fiscal, and patient outcomes related to a research-based change. This step is essential in determining the effectiveness of both the practice change and the strategies used for implementation of the guidelines. It is also the most difficult step because baseline measures may be limited or absent. For example, prior to implementation of the pain scales and the Braden Scale (Braden, 1989), no standardized tools were in place to collect these data routinely at UIHC. When data were routinely collected without standardized tools, validity was questionable. Both skin breakdown and inadequately controlled pain were underreported.

Incorporation of the guidelines into care maps has addressed these limitations and greatly enhanced the ability to measure patient outcomes. Standardized assessment tools are used, evaluation is completed on a routine basis, and variances are analyzed and trends indentified. Cost of variances can be calculated. For example, an increased length of stay related to skin breakdown is readily identified as a variance.

For patients not included in the case management program, outcomes are monitored through risk management and quality improvement (QI) activities at the hospital, department, and unit level. Routinely collected risk management data about incidence of skin breakdown have been enhanced and can be compared to the level of risk identified for individual patients on the admission assessment form and the interventions used. This provides a more valid evaluation of patient care. Pain management activities have also been evaluated using QI data. Baseline data have been collected on every inpatient nursing unit, including data on the level of most severe pain experienced during a 24-hour period and satisfaction with pain management. When postimplementation data were compared to this baseline, results were very positive. Before changes in pain management, 68% of obstetrics and gynecology patients reported pain ratings of 3 or less on a 1 to 10 scale. After pain assessment and management were enhanced on care maps, these low ratings were reported by 90% of this patient population. And the results were replicated hospital-wide: 41% more critical care patients reported low pain ratings after implementation of the guideline. Patients in the Surgical Nursing/Cancer Center Division reported significant reductions in pain and increased satisfaction with pain management after round-the-clock dosing of analgesics.

Skin integrity is also measured throughout the nursing department. When the Braden Scale (1989) was implemented, nurses' awareness of skin integrity was heightened, and more referrals were made to the enterostomal therapy nurse. Thus more patients are receiving early intervention rather than risking progression to more serious skin breakdown.

Along with patient outcomes, data are being collected about the processes used to implement the guidelines and the impact on staff. For example, in Pediatrics, nurses are being surveyed to determine their knowledge level, attitudes toward pain management, and satisfaction with the change process (Schmidt et al., 1994). This information can be used to plan future educational programs for staff, as well as to plan additional changes to facilitate use of the guidelines in practice.

In addition to evaluating the impact of clinical practice guidelines within an institution, it is important for nurse administrators to provide feedback about the impact of guidelines on patient outcomes to the AHCPR (American Hospital Association, 1992). This information will be used for future revision of the guidelines, ensuring that interventions included are clinically achievable and result in positive patient outcomes.

SUMMARY

Clinical practice guidelines provide a thorough, relevant review of multidisciplinary treatment options for selected patient problems. The concise, easy-to-read format minimized some barriers to utilizing research findings in practice—those barriers associated with the research and communication. However, the most frequently identified barriers are associated with the setting and must be addressed by the nurse administrator. Mechanisms used to minimize these barriers and successful strategies for implementation of the guidelines in a large teaching hospital have been presented by using the Iowa model (Titler et al., 1994). The results have been positive for both patients and staff. The quality of patient care has been standardized at a higher level of quality, consistent with available knowledge. Also, nurses report feeling empowered by a research-based practice and the ability to discuss alternatives for patient care with physicians.

NOTE

1. Information about clinical practice guidelines can be obtained by contacting the U.S. Department of Health and Human Services, Public Health Services, Agency for Health Care Policy and Research, Rockville, MD, 20852, 1-(800)-358-9295.

REFERENCES

Acute Pain Management Guideline Panel. (1992a). *Acute pain management: Operative or medical procedures and trauma* (AHCPR Pub No. 92-0032). Rockville, MD: Agency for Health Care Policy and Research, Public Health Service, U.S. Dept. of Health and Human Services.

Acute Pain Management Guideline Panel. (1992b). *Acute pain management in infants, children, and adolescents: Operative or medical procedures* (AHCPR Pub No. 92-0020). Rockville, MD: Agency for Health Care Policy and Research, Public Health Service, U.S. Dept. of Health and Human Services.

American Hospital Association. (1992, September). *CPG strategies: Putting guidelines into practice.* Chicago: Author.

Benign Prostatic Hyperplasia Guideline Panel. (1994). *Benign prostatic hyperplasia: Diagnosis and treatment* (AHCPR Pub No. 94-0582). Rockville, MD: Agency for Health Care Policy and Research, Public Health Service, U.S. Dept. of Health and Human Services.

Braden, B. (1989). Clinical utility of the Braden Scale for predicting pressure sore risk. *Decubitus, 2*(3), 44-6, 50-1.

Cataract Management Guideline Panel. (1993). *Cataract in adults: Management of functional impairment* (AHCPR Pub No. 93-0542). Rockville, MD: Agency for Health Care Policy and Research, Public Health Service, U.S. Dept. of Health and Human Services.

Champion, V., & Leach, A. (1989). Variables related to research utilization in nursing: An empirical investigation. *Journal of Advanced Nursing, 14,* 705-710.

Depression Guideline Panel. (1993). *Depression in primary care: Vol. 1. Detection and diagnosis* (AHCPR Pub. No. 93-0550). Rockville, MD: Agency for Health Care Policy and Research, Public Health Service, U.S. Dept. of Health and Human Services.

Funk, S., Champagne, M., Wiess, R., & Tournquist, E. (1991). Barriers to using research findings in practice: The clinician's perspective. *Applied Nursing Research, 4*(2), 90-95.

Goode, C., & Bulechek, G. (1992). Research utilization: An organizational process that enhances quality of care. *Journal of Nursing Care Quality, 6,* 27-35.

Kraus, V., Fink, L., Hradek, E., & Sueppel, C. (1994). *Agency for Health Care Policy and Research (AHCPR) and clinical practice guidelines: An instructional packet.* Iowa City: University of Iowa Hospitals and Clinics.

Management of Cancer Pain Guideline Panel. (1994). *Management of cancer pain* (AHCPR Pub. No. 94-0592). Rockville, MD: Agency for Health Care Policy and Research, Public Health Service, U.S. Dept. of Health and Human Services.

Miller, J., & Messenger, S. (1978). Obstacles to applying nursing research findings. *American Journal of Nursing, 78,* 632-634.

Panel for the Prediction and Prevention of Pressure Ulcers in Adults. (1992). *Pressure ulcers in adults: Prediction and prevention* (AHCPR Pub. No. 92-0047). Rockville, MD: Agency for Health Care Policy and Research, Public Health Service, U.S. Dept. of Health and Human Services.

Pettengill, M., Gillies, D., & Clark, C. (1994). Factors encouraging and discouraging the use of nursing research findings. *Image, 26,* 143-147.

Schmidt, K., Holida, D., Kleiber, C., Peterson, M., & Phearman, L. (1994). Implementation of AHCPR pain guidelines for children. *Journal of Nursing Care Quality, 8*(3), 68-74.

Sickle Cell Disease Guideline Panel. (1993). *Sickle cell disease: Screening, diagnosis, management, and counseling in newborns and infants* (AHCPR Pub. No. 93-0562). Rockville, MD: Agency for Health Care Policy and Research, Public Health Service, U.S. Dept. of Health and Human Services.

Titler, M., Kleiber, C., Steelman, V., Goode, C., Rakel, B., Barry-Walker, J., Small, S., & Buckwalter, K. (1994). Infusing research into practice to promote quality care. *Nursing Research, 43,* 307-313.

Urinary Incontinence Guideline Panel. (1992). *Urinary incontinence in adults* (AHCPR Pub. No. 92-0038). Rockville, MD: Agency for Health Care Policy and Research, Public Health Service, U.S. Dept. of Health and Human Services.

CHAPTER 9

The Impact of a Creative Staffing Schedule on Nursing Practice at an Academic Medical Center

Jean A. Walters

The purposes of nurse scheduling models are to provide maximum flexibility for nursing staff with their desired schedules while enhancing patient care delivery. The 7/70 scheduling model at Froedtert Hospital in Milwaukee is based on three overlapping 10-hour shifts, with nurses working one of three overlapping 10-hour shifts every other week for 7 days, then having the following week off. Seven hours of overlap occur with this scheduling model, allowing nurses time to carry out complex nursing care routines, professional activities, and patient education. The cost-effectiveness of 7/70 scheduling was evaluated prior to its implementation when the hospital opened 14 years ago and is evaluated on an ongoing basis. A recent study has shown that the cost of our 7/70 schedule remains very favorable when compared with nursing hours provided at other institutions. In 1992 nursing surveys at Froedtert, 7/70 scheduling was unequivocally indicated as the number one reason that nurses choose to work at Froedtert Hospital and the number one reason nurses remain at Froedtert. The 7/70 RN turnover rates are well within norms for urban teaching hospitals. Nurses are not the only individuals who are satisfied with the impact of 7/70. Physicians and patients are pleased with the continuity of care provided to patients by the 7/70 nursing staff. This scheduling, however, tends to attract a younger nurse than national average. Because our nurses are young and often join us as new graduates, we have few nurses with advanced degrees and experience in nursing research. A number of steps have therefore been implemented to promote nursing research. Despite the many advantages of 7/70 scheduling, a few nurses who have worked 7/70 for some time have expressed a desire for a less rigorous schedule. Although 7/70 will remain our primary scheduling model, we are currently investigating other innovative schedules to assess their fit with staff and patient needs. Despite a few disadvantages, the 7/70 scheduling model has many benefits for nurses, physicians, patients, and administration and has been deemed highly successful.

Staff nurse scheduling has remained the bane of nurse managers over the years. It is a constant challenge to balance patient needs with available nursing staff. According to Stumpf (1989), the goals of a scheduling system are to ensure an adequate number and appropriate type of nursing personnel on each shift and day to meet predetermined nursing hours, to balance the needs of patients with the needs of staff, to distribute fairly the assignment of less desirable shifts, to provide advance posting of the schedules to all staff to plan their personal lives, to provide a mechanism to accommodate emergency changes, to provide continuity of care, and to conform with labor laws. It remains a challenge to meet all these goals, and attempts to do so have resulted in the implementation of many creative staffing schedules over the past 20 years. The ultimate goal of these unique staffing schedules is to provide maximum flexibility for nursing staff while enhancing patient care delivery. Although the impact of creative staffing schedules should be positive, inevitably there are a few disadvantages to innovative staffing schedules. The purpose of this chapter is to discuss one innovative schedule, a 7/70 scheduling model at Froedtert Memorial Lutheran Hospital, a 295-bed, academic, tertiary medical center in Milwaukee, Wisconsin, and its impact on the cost of providing care, RN recruitment and retention, the amount of nursing research conducted, and physician and patient satisfaction.

7/70 SCHEDULING MODEL

The 7/70 scheduling model (7 consecutive 10-hour days, equaling a total of 70 hours in a 2-week pay period) was conceived and first implemented at Evergreen General Hospital, Kirkland, Washington, in 1972 (Hutchins & Cleveland, 1978). Subsequently, it was implemented at several hospitals in the Pacific Northwest, in Indiana, and at Froedtert Memorial Lutheran Hospital when it opened in 1980.

This scheduling model is based on three overlapping 10-hour shifts. RNs are scheduled to work one of three overlapping 10-hour shifts every other week for 7 days, Monday through Sunday (Figure 9.1). RNs then have the following

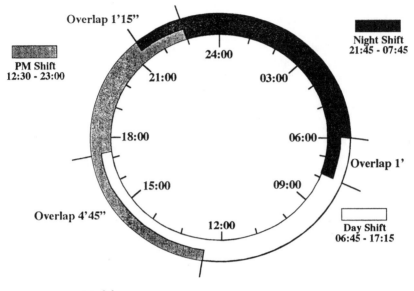

Figure 9.1. 7/70 Workday

week off while another team of nurses works its week of three overlapping 10-hour shifts. The shift times are:

First shift	6:45 a.m. to 5:15 p.m. (10.5 hrs.)
Second shift	12:30 p.m. to 11:00 p.m. (10.5 hrs.)
Third shift	9:45 p.m. to 7:45 a.m. (10 hrs.)

The third shift is only 10 hours due to RNs' inability to leave the floor for a half-hour uninterrupted lunch break. Therefore staff use their shorter breaks to eat quick meals.

RNs in intensive care and acute care units work this 7/70 scheduling system. The nursing manager, called the patient care director (PCD), works a traditional 10/80 scheduling system (10 eight-hour shifts in a 2-week pay period, equaling a total of 80 hours) and is a link to maintaining communication and continuity of patient care between the two teams of nurses.

In addition to the nursing department, other departments have adopted the 7/70 scheduling system, if appropriate to meet their staff and service needs. Mariella Larter (1982), the first Vice President of Patient Care Services at Froedtert in 1980, defined the essentials of the 7/70 scheduling system as follows:

1. The department must be open 24 hours per day on a 7-day-per-week basis.
2. There are three overlapping 10-hour shifts.
3. Staff are paid for the 70 hours worked but receive benefits on a full-time basis.

These essentials helped identify which departments, nursing and non-nursing, could work a 7/70 schedule. The clinical systems communicators (unit clerks) work a modified 7/70 schedule with a 10-hour day and night shift and a 5-hour evening shift. Some Respiratory Therapy and Pharmacy staff also work a modified 7/70 schedule. RNs in Surgery, Post-Anesthesia Care Unit (PACU), clinics, and other areas work more traditional scheduling systems. Not all 7/70 staff have to work full time. Two 7/70 staff may work part time and "job-share," one working 3 days of the 7-day work week and the other working 4 days. This 3-day/4-day rotation may be reversed every other work week if staff desire.

Upon hire, each nurse is assigned to either one Monday to Sunday week (A Week) or the following Monday to Sunday week (B Week), with no shift rotation. Three of the 10-hour shifts fall on one payroll work week and four in the next. Froedtert's 2-week work cycle begins on a Friday and ends on a Thursday. Staff are able to work an additional 10 hours, beyond the 70-hour work week, in their 30-hour week and be paid at their base rate. Staff receive overtime for any extra hours worked during their 40-hour work week.

OVERLAP

The 7/70 scheduling model for RNs allows 7 hours of overlap in a 24-hour day ($4\frac{3}{4}$ hours in the early p.m., $1\frac{1}{4}$ hour in the late p.m., and 1 hour in the early a.m.). To equalize the pace of activity and minimize nurse fatigue in a 7/70 model, heavy nursing care tasks are planned during the overlap hours. In addition, professional activities, patient education, patient conferences, continuous quality improvement, and other activities are carried out during overlap.

PRIMARY NURSING

To further enhance the continuity of care at Froedtert, a primary nursing model is utilized. The primary nurse assignment is determined among the nurses on each unit. Froedtert has many repeat patients, and nurses who have been a primary nurse for a patient during a previous hospitalization are able to take their past patient as a primary for subsequent hospital stays. If patient stays exceed the nurse's 7-day work week, a coprimary nurse is determined for the alternate week. Associate nurses continue the continuity of care for the 14 hours of each day when the primary or coprimary nurse is not on duty. This combination of 7/70 scheduling with primary nursing truly enhances continuity of patient care.

LITERATURE REVIEW ON 7/70 SCHEDULES

Few current articles on the 7/70 scheduling model are found. This may be because 7/70 is perceived to be more costly in today's cost-conscious health care economy. Andron and Hunter (1988) wrote about the use of a 7/70 scheduling system in a laboratory setting. Although the nursing examples of 7/70 scheduling are not recent, they will be reviewed in this chapter for background information.

Dison, Carter, and Bromley (1981) indicated that many nursing administrators first began to utilize flexible scheduling options, such as 7/70, 5/40, and 12-hour shifts, to reduce the cost of agency staff utilization. At Baptist Hospital in Miami, a nursing survey was conducted to identify problems with the existing scheduling system (Dison et al., 1981). This survey indicated 46% dissatisfaction with the amount of RN control in planning the work schedule. Gulack (1982) reported on an RN magazine survey on RN preferences regarding scheduling options. He reported that 6 of 10 part-time RNs would work full time if they could work over 8 hours in a day.

The results of the 7/70 scheduling model, as reported in past literature, are primarily positive. Dison et al. (1981) reported that South Miami Hospital, which utilized a variety of schedules, including 7/70, decreased agency utilization, increased success in RN recruitment, and increased nursing staff satisfaction and stability with its flexible scheduling. They reported that the higher cost for flexible scheduling was offset by reduced use of agency staff.

At institutions utilizing primarily 7/70 scheduling, such as Group Health Hospital in Redmond, Oregon, results were that the 7/70 schedule resolved coverage problems during overlap, reduced nurse fatigue, and increased continuity of care and staff communication. Group Health Hospital reported that nurses loved every other week off and appreciated the reduced transportation and child care costs. RNs felt more rested after their week off and had high morale (Donovan, 1978). Rabideau and Skarbek (1978) reported that the biggest benefit of 7/70 was the improvement in patient care. Other benefits reported were that patients liked the continuity of knowing who would be taking care of them each day and that staff assessments of patient needs were more thorough and accurate. In addition, the same nurses working together for 7 days resulted in friendships as well as professional collegiality. The 7/70 schedule also created a better rapport between physicians and RNs. The disadvantages of 7/70, however, were that RNs lost approximately one eighth of their income and were fatigued at the end of the 7-day work week. This fatigue, however, was eliminated after a night of good rest. In addition, Rabideau and Skarbek reported less use of sick time because staff were less susceptible to illness with every other week off. An *American Journal of Nursing* article ("The Demise of the Traditional 5-40 Workweek?" 1981) reported on problems with 7/70 at Valley Medical Center in Fresno, California. This article indicated a lack of continuity with the complete change of shift every 7 days. Valley Medical Center countered this lack of continuity by having the nursing manager work a traditional staffing schedule and be the communication link between the 2 weeks. One unanticipated benefit of 7/70 at Valley Medical Center was a marked improvement in documentation due to the increased improvement of written information on patient status necessary for communication between the 2 weeks.

Hutchins and Cleveland (1978) reported that overlap was used for lunch, report, finishing complicated care, patient education, charting, counting narcotics, and in-services. Staff liked taking full, uninterrupted lunches and being able to relax, knowing that their patients were well cared for. Staff also reported not going home feeling rushed, as if they had forgotten something.

Andron and Hunter (1988) reported on a 7/70 schedule implemented in a hospital laboratory. Staff were scheduled to work seven consecutive 10-hour days followed by a 7-day break. The pay period ran from Sunday through Saturday. The 7/70 work week began on a Thursday. By scheduling 30 hours in one pay period and 40 hours in the other, "artificial" overtime was eliminated. Andron and Hunter reported that this 7/70 scheduling plan boosted morale, increased productivity, and decreased staff burnout. In addition, some staff worked extra on their week off, making filling of relief for sick and vacation time easier. Andron and Hunter indicated, however, that not all staff preferred 7/70 scheduling.

LITERATURE REVIEW ON
OTHER SCHEDULING MODELS

A variety of work schedules are reported in the current literature, with 12-hour shifts being the most predominant. Donovan (1978) reported on the 4-day, 40-hour week at Roger Williams General Hospital in Providence, Rhode Island. The results of this 4/40 schedule were inadequate overlap of teams from day to day, RN fatigue at the end of the shift, problems in recruiting staff for a permanent p.m. shift, and staff who either loved or hated the schedule. Donovan also reported that this 4/40 scheduling was not cost-effective because it paid the RN 10 hours of sick pay rather than 8. Eventually, the hospital dropped this 4/40 model because of staff and overlap problems.

Numerous articles indicated the benefits and drawbacks of 12-hour schedules. Slota and Balas-Stevens (1990) reported that a changeover to 12-hour shifts created an increase in RN creativity, an increase in autonomy, innovation in the work environment, a decrease in RN turnover rates, a decrease in staff physical and emotional problems, no change in job satisfaction, no increase in errors, less clarity regarding daily routines, and more communication problems. Overall, however, Slota and Balas-Stevens reported a positive impact for 12-hour shifts. Other benefits of 12-hour shifts perceived by RNs included fewer days on duty; less staff commuting time; safer traveling times; decreased staff sick time; closer rapport with the patient, the patient's significant others, and other staff; improved communication between shifts; and an ability to meet the patient's needs more adequately. Lillis (1989) added the following advantages of 12-hour shifts: fewer staff required, lower costs per patient day, and less friction among staff due to having only two shifts rather than three. Despite all of these advantages, 12-hour shifts do have the following disadvantages: increased mental exhaustion and tension after shifts; decreased quality of staff days off; a lack of continuity of patient care, with staff working a few days on followed by more days off; and an insufficient amount of overlap time necessary for report and other vital communications. Houston (1990) added the disadvantages of less flexibility in scheduling within a 40-hour work week and longer time away from family on work days.

The literature is divided regarding the overall impact of 12-hour shifts; however, Gowell and Boverie (1992) found that 10-hour shifts were preferred to 8- and 12-hour shifts. In addition, Velianoff (1991) reported that a 10-hour shift entailed less drudgery than a 12-hour shift and that after a trial, 90% of staff preferred a 10-hour shift to a 12-hour shift.

COST-EFFECTIVENESS OF 7/70 SCHEDULING

The cost-effectiveness of the Froedtert 7/70 scheduling model was evaluated prior to its implementation when the hospital opened 14 years ago and continues to be evaluated on an ongoing basis as the health care financial environment changes. Larter (1982) reported on how a 7/70 nursing budget was projected, using an average occupancy of 22 patients for a 26-bed unit with a 5-hours-of-care-per-patient-day requirement:

Bed capacity of unit	26 beds
Average occupancy	22 patients
Required nursing workforce	$22 \times 5 = 110$ hours
Personnel required for an 8-hour shift	$110 \div 8 = 13.75$ people
Personnel required for a 10-hour shift	$110 \div 10 = 11$ people

The master schedule showed the utilization of the above staff in both the traditional and 7/70 schedules:

	Day Shift	Evening Shift	Night Shift
Traditional system	6	5	3
7/70 system	4	4	3

Total budget preparation for a 7/70 schedule is identical to that of a typical schedule, with the difference found merely in the application of the allocated hours at the nursing unit level. Our budget formula is:

$$\text{Budgeted Manhours for Unit} \times \text{Budgeted Average Daily Census for Unit} \times 365 \text{ days/yr.} \div 2{,}080 \text{ hours}$$

This formula gives the number of productive RN Full Time Equivalencies (FTEs) from which the unit's core staffing is derived. A nonproductive percentage is added to the productive FTEs for the unit's total FTE component. The budget preparation for the above unit would be created thus:

$$5 \times 22 \times 365 \div 2{,}800 = 19.3 \text{ FTEs}$$

To convert these 2,080 FTEs to 7/70 FTEs (with 1,820 hrs.), the following formula is used:

$$19.3 \times 2{,}080 \div 1{,}820 = 22.05 \text{ FTEs available for core staffing}$$

A nonproductive factor is added to the 2,080 FTE number to get the total FTEs for the unit budget.

$$19.3 \ (2{,}080) \text{ FTEs} \times 10\% \text{ nonproductive factor} = 21.2 \ (2{,}080) \text{ FTEs}$$

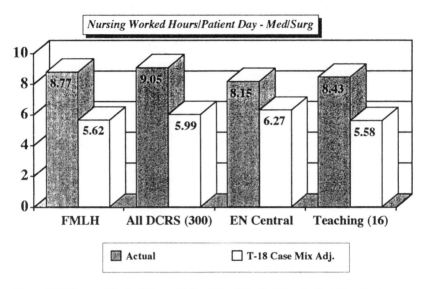

Figure 9.2. Nursing Worked Hours/Patient Day (Medical/Surgical) at Froedtert Versus Other Voluntary Hospitals of America, Data Comparison Reporting System (DCRS), 1992 Data

Therefore the total number of FTEs available to cover total hours for this unit, both staffing and nonproductive hours, is 21.2.

In summary, the PCD prepares the budget as if staff were 2,080 hour staff (i.e., "traditional FTEs") and converts these "traditional" FTEs to 7/70 FTEs for scheduling purposes. The PCD, however, is held to compliance with the "traditional" 2,080 FTE salary projection compared with the actual average daily census. The FTE salary dollars are flexed up or down each month with the actual census statistics. This "flexed" salary dollar is then compared with the unit's "actual" salary dollar to determine salary compliance. Therefore, although the PCD converts staff to a 7/70 schedule, the PCD is held accountable to keep actual salary dollars within the traditional 2,080 FTE flexed salary dollars.

To validate further the cost-effectiveness of our 7/70 scheduling, comparative data have been evaluated. A recent study has shown that the cost of our 7/70 nursing schedule remains very favorable when compared with nursing hours provided at other institutions. The Data Comparison Reporting System (DCRS) from the Voluntary Hospitals of America (VHA) and the Monitrend Report from the American Hospital Association have indicated that the nursing hours delivered in our 7/70 scheduling model are very comparable with those

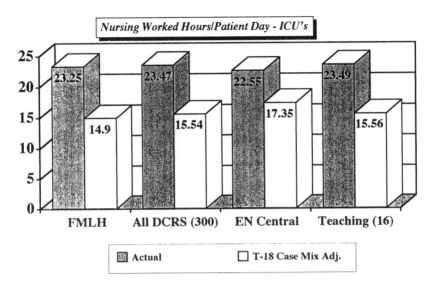

Figure 9.3. Nursing Worked Hours/Patient Day (ICU) at Froedtert Versus Other Voluntary Hospitals of America, Data Comparison Reporting System (DCRS), 1992 Data

provided at other hospitals (data adjusted for case mix index and comparative personnel costs; see Figures 9.2 through 9.4).

Although the costs for actual nursing hours delivered are very favorable, one additional cost must be factored in to determine the total cost of our 7/70 scheduling system. Staff working 7/70 full time (i.e., 70 hours in a pay period) receive full-time benefits. At Froedtert, 256 RNs now work 7/70. If the scheduling system used 2,080 FTEs, only 224 FTEs would be necessary. Therefore we are paying an "additional" 32 staff full-time benefits with our 7/70 system. The fringe benefits and paid time off for these 32 staff cost the hospital $189,350. This is a substantial investment for an institution, but this cost must be countered with the positive benefits received in the areas of RN retention and recruitment.

Another significant cost and quality benefit due to the 7/70 scheduling system has been that the hospital is one of only two hospitals in the Milwaukee area that have never used agency staff for supplemental RN staffing. The 7/70 staff are available to work extra on their week off, and many choose to work one or more extra shifts to increase their pay to 80 or more hours per pay period. This willingness of staff to work extra on their week off increases the

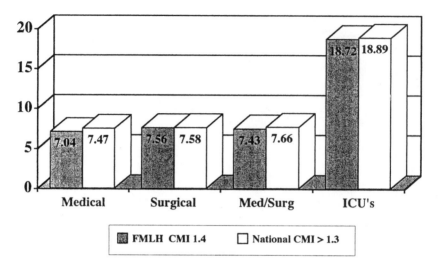

Figure 9.4. Nursing Worked Hours/Patient Day at Froedtert Versus Other American Hospital Association Hospitals, Monitrend Reporting System, 1992 Data

hospital's ease in flexing up to meet staffing needs. The fact that Froedtert has never used outside agency RNs for staffing has contributed significantly to reducing the impact of the cost of providing full-time benefits for 7/70 staff. In addition, it has a very positive impact on the quality of nursing care provided.

In summary, 7/70 promotes the quality of nursing care because it retains staff experienced in Froedtert's tertiary care and has eliminated the need to use supplemental agency RNs for staffing. These facts justify the additional cost of the benefits provided to 7/70 staff.

IMPACT OF 7/70 ON
RN RECRUITMENT AND RETENTION

In 1992, data were gathered from all RNs newly employed at Froedtert. These data indicated that 7/70 scheduling was unequivocally the number one reason RNs chose to work at Froedtert. When we recently asked Milwaukee area hospitals for major factors that recruited RNs to their hospital, no other hospital indicated a scheduling model as a main recruitment factor. This comparison indicates that 7/70 definitely gives Froedtert a competitive advantage over other area hospitals.

RESPONSES:

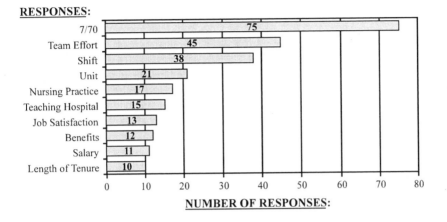

Figure 9.5. Top-Ranked Responses to Question "What Single Factor Retains You at Froedtert?" (1992 Nursing Survey Data From RNs Newly Employed at Froedtert)

The impact of 7/70 on RN retention is just as striking as the impact on recruitment. A 1992 survey was also completed with RNs then currently employed at Froedtert. Two hundred and four RNs (42% return rate) responded to the survey. According to this survey, the 7/70 scheduling model was also the major factor that retained nurses (Figure 9.5). To further validate which factors retain staff, we asked the respondents the open-ended question, "What single factor works well at Froedtert?" The 7/70 schedule again led as the outstanding factor that worked well. The positive impact of 7/70 can be seen in several other responses in Figure 9.5. Group teamwork, overlap use, and team effort were ranked high as factors that retained staff and that worked well. Hostility between shifts is much less apt to occur when there is a significant overlap time and two teams are working side by side for hours at a time. The fact that one shift of staff can go to lunch together also enhances the sociability of the group.

Another positive impact of 7/70 can be seen in the sick rate. Data for 1993 at Froedtert indicated that non-7/70 RNs who worked in traditional areas such as Surgery and Clinics used an average of 5.6 eight-hour shifts of sick time (or 45.03 average sick hours per RN), whereas 7/70 RNs used an average of 4.7 ten-hour shifts of sick time (or 47.29 average sick hours per RN). Although the total sick hours per RN are slightly higher for 7/70 staff, this may be a function of how staff sick incidents occur. Usually staff feel ill and call in before the beginning of a shift rather than leave midshift. Therefore 7/70 staff receive pay for a 10-hour shift, whereas non-7/70 staff receive pay for an 8-hour shift. This sick day payment policy could be changed to reduce 7/70 sick day payments to 8 hours, which would lower total costs for 7/70 sick hours. The fact that fewer 7/70 10-hour "sick day" shifts needed to be replaced in 1993 should also be considered. In addition, 7/70 shifts can be replaced with a partial shift, due to the RN overlap that exists with 7/70, thus reducing the cost of replacing 7/70 sick shifts. In summary, although the average sick hours of 7/70 staff are not dramatically different from those of non-7/70 staff, this is partly due to staff's use of sick time and the sick day payment policy. In addition, the replacement cost is reduced because the overlap planned in the 7/70 schedule permits partial shift replacement without compromising quality.

The 7/70 RN turnover rates have also been low in the past and are well within norms for urban teaching hospitals. In addition, many RNs who leave the hospital for "greener pastures" or other reasons return to employment at Froedtert at a later date. This return rate also helps to validate that 7/70 is important, as it is a factor often mentioned by returning staff. The fact that 7/70 is a major retention strategy has been validated recently by concerns raised during a change in top hospital administration. A new president had been hired, and the major concern of the nursing staff for months before and after the new president's hire was whether 7/70 would change.

The positive impact of 7/70 was recently highlighted by one nurse in an article on 7/70 in the Froedtert Hospital Newsletter. The RN reported that because nurses were at the hospital for 7 days in a row, it was much easier to see patient progression or regression and subtle differences in patients from day to day. The nurse concluded that 7/70 offered the best of both worlds, making it easier for her to be both a mother and a nurse and that it was easy to plan family activities because she could always know when she would have time off. These comments help to capture many of the feelings of RNs working 7/70 at Froedtert and reinforce why 7/70 RNs remain at Froedtert.

IMPACT OF 7/70 ON TYPE OF
NURSE EMPLOYED AT FROEDTERT

The 7/70 scheduling plan at Froedtert tends to attract a younger nurse than the national standard. Froedtert attracts a larger number of young staff for a variety of reasons. Its affiliation with many schools of nursing in the Milwaukee area exposes many student nurses to our environment. Its nurse extern program allows student nurses to be employed with an expanded patient care assistant role. Many of these student nurses and nurse externs become employed at Froedtert upon graduation. Also, young experienced nurses are attracted to Froedtert because of its specialization, its state-of-the-art nursing and medical practice, and the fact that it is an academic medical center. Because working a 70-hour week requires a certain amount of physical stamina, 7/70 is more attractive to younger nurses. The perception of RNs outside Froedtert is that 7/70 is physically challenging. However, after several weeks of working 7/70, most staff report that they have adjusted to the intensive schedule. This perception of 7/70 as physically challenging tends to demotivate older nurses from working 7/70.

Froedtert nurses are younger than the national average, and many join Froedtert as graduate nurses. Although 41% of our staff are baccalaureate prepared, few have their master's degree. Therefore fewer nurses at Froedtert have experience in nursing research. Although many staff use the tuition reimbursement policy to continue their education and may thereby utilize nursing research, enhancing RN utilization of the nursing research process remains a challenge to nursing administration, which recognizes its value in enhancing professionalism and practice. Therefore a number of steps have been taken to encourage nursing research at Froedtert. First, Froedtert initiated a contract with a local university for the part-time services of a PhD-prepared nurse researcher. This researcher attends all Nursing Research Committee meetings, gives direction to the nursing research effort at Froedtert, and, most important, is on site a half day each week to assist any interested nurse in working through the nursing research process. This on-site, one-on-one assistance has proven invaluable to staff nurses who are interested in researching an idea. The Nursing Research Committee, assisted by this individual, has made annual efforts to encourage nurses to use her services, with increasing success every year.

Another effort that has proven very successful was implemented several years ago. Nursing administration felt that if financial support were available, more nurses would participate in the nursing research process. Therefore a request was made to the Froedtert Auxiliary to fund a nursing research grant that would make annual research dollars available to Froedtert nursing staff. The auxiliary graciously funded a grant large enough to make annual monies available to nursing staff from the interest generated on the principal grant amount. To make this grant even more effective, one criterion for obtaining the grant is that nurses who are new to the nursing research process are given first preference. That does not mean that the standards for a quality nursing research proposal and project are lowered, only that if two research proposals are equal, the nurse without nursing research experience will be given preference. To ensure the quality of proposals submitted by nurses new to the research process, staff are strongly encouraged to seek out the services of our PhD-prepared nursing researcher. The first year that the grant was available, four nurses new to the research process were recipients of the grant. Over the past 2 years, eight nurses new to the research process and seven nurses experienced in nursing research have been recipients of $6,235 through the grant, thereby increasing RN involvement in nursing research at Froedtert.

Froedtert has also sought to involve actively nurses not familiar with the research process in a formal nursing research project through participation on a task force conducting nursing research. In 1989, nursing administration, with the guidance of the PhD-prepared nursing researcher, sought to create a valid and reliable tool with which to measure the severity of medication errors. A task force consisting of nurses new to and nurses familiar with the research process reviewed the literature and existing medication error severity tools and were involved in the creation of a tool. The task force also determined the validity and reliability of the new tool. The tool was piloted and eventually implemented in our hospital. In taking the research project one step further, staff nurses from this task force were invited to be coauthors of an article about the process and its results. This involvement in publication was received with interest and enthusiasm by all invited, and subsequently several staff nurses who had previously not been involved in any research were involved in research and became coauthors of a published article on this process (Walters et al., 1992).

Froedtert's continuous quality improvement program (QUEST) also helps to identify opportunities in which nursing research and QUEST can be combined. One example was a study completed by operating room staff to determine if sterilized items were no longer sterile upon the item's outdate. Staff's research found that sterilized articles with no tear or opening in the wrapping remained sterile. These findings reduced hospital expenses by $10,000 annually (O'Connor, 1994; Schroeter, 1994). The Nursing Research Committee is currently attempting to make nursing staff more aware of the similarities between QUEST and the nursing research process in an effort to make nursing research less intimidating for nursing staff. An article was written for the nursing research newsletter on such similarities, highlighting studies such as the OR sterility project. The quality improvement director also helps the Nursing Research Committee identify appropriate QUEST projects that could become research studies.

Despite the disadvantage of a younger 7/70 staff without much experience in nursing research, Froedtert's efforts to encourage nursing research enhances RN professionalism and promotes the quality of nursing care provided. In addition, Froedtert's younger staff bring enthusiasm and interest to nursing research. This makes staff more open to learning about and using the nursing research process and its results.

IMPACT OF 7/70 ON PHYSICIAN SATISFACTION

Physicians have always felt that a high quality of nursing care is provided at Froedtert. In the past, physicians have been very pleased with the continuity of care provided by RNs working the 7/70 scheduling model. This perception has recently been validated in a 1993 physician survey. Fifty-five physicians were interviewed to gather data on ways to enhance MD/RN collaboration. Results indicated that the closer the physician worked directly with the nurse at the bedside, the more the physician noted the benefits of 7/70. Although the vast majority of physician respondents did indicate a positive value to 7/70, a few physicians had no strong feelings or felt there was little benefit with 7/70 and that it did not help with MD/RN collaboration. Overall, however, the vast majority of MDs surveyed were supportive of 7/70. Some of their comments were:

- 7/70 is very beneficial due to the continuity of patient care related to RNs' knowledge of patients (treatments, status and plan of care).
- MDs seldom hear "I do not know this patient. I just picked the patient up" from the RNs.
- 7/70 RNs seemed to become personally involved in patient care because of better awareness of patient status.
- MDs enjoy working with the same nurse over an extended period of time.
- It is easy for the MD to determine which nurse has which patient.
- 7/70 engenders RN loyalty to the hospital.
- 7/70 has the potential to decrease RN burnout and increase overall positive attitudes.

Therefore results of the physician surveys support physicians' satisfaction with the 7/70 scheduling model.

IMPACT OF 7/70 ON PATIENT SATISFACTION

Patients have traditionally been very satisfied with the nursing care at Froedtert Hospital, frequently commenting on the fact that they have gotten to know their nurse and been very pleased with the coordination of their care during hospitalization. Focus groups of former Froedtert patients indicated only glowing reports about the nursing care. Some focus group participants mentioned that they really liked having the same nurse for a week; this indicates a positive response to 7/70. The nurses seemed to come to mind first when the participants judged the quality of their stay at the hospital. Participants in the focus groups mentioned how the nurses seemed like family after a while at Froedtert. The level of personal care and concern by nurses was said to be excellent. The nurses took the time to listen to patients, talk with them, and answer questions. All participants felt that the nurses at Froedtert knew what they were doing.

To further validate this perception of patient satisfaction with the continuity of nursing care, Froedtert recently participated in a national comparative study of patient satisfaction with hospital care (Table 9.1). Of the 200 Froedtert participants in the sample, 95 completed surveys for a 48% response rate. Although the questions asked in this comparative study do not directly relate to the 7/70 scheduling system, the overall results of the study indicated that the nursing care provided is at a high level and definitely promotes quality patient care.

FUTURE PLANS

It is the intent of the hospital to keep the cost of providing nursing care at as cost-effective a level as possible. To that end, the cost of using the 7/70 scheduling system has been closely evaluated in the past and will continue to be closely evaluated in the future. This evaluation, however, must consider not only all of the costs but all of the benefits derived from 7/70. In any nursing care provision environment, many opportunities for reducing costs exist. Froedtert is currently evaluating opportunities to reduce costs throughout the organization, and it is possible that 7/70 may be modified in some way. However, because of the many benefits that 7/70 brings to RN, patient, and physician satisfaction, and because it eliminates the use of supplemental agency staffing, it is anticipated that the basic framework will remain, with some modifications to enhance cost-effectiveness. One disadvantage of 7/70 previously indicated is that it is physically taxing and therefore appeals to younger individuals. Because Froedtert is now 14 years old, a number of nursing staff have been with the hospital since its opening. Some staff would not trade 7/70 for anything. A few, however, are interested in alternative scheduling models such as 8- and 12-hour shifts. Interspersing these alternative shifts with 7/70 will eliminate overlap hours and reduce costs. This is one way that the costs for providing nursing care in a 7/70 schedule can be reduced. Other such avenues will be pursued in the near future to enhance cost savings for RN staffing.

TABLE 9.1   Overall Opinion of Nursing Care Results From 1993 National Patient
Survey

Rating	Froedtert	Average Facility
Excellent	75%	68%
Good	22%	27%
Total	97%	95%

NOTE: N = 95 or 48% response rate.

SUMMARY

This chapter has analyzed the impact of an innovative scheduling model, 7/70, on the costs of providing nursing care, RN recruitment and retention, the amount of nursing research conducted, and physician and patient satisfaction. Despite a few disadvantages, the 7/70 scheduling model has many benefits for nurses, physicians, patients, and administration and has been deemed highly successful. In the future, nursing administrators must continue to work closely with nursing staff to create scheduling models that promote both quality patient care and cost-effectiveness. The health care industry will need to be open to flexibility and creativity in future approaches to staff scheduling.

The 7/70 staff scheduling model is one creative scheduling model and is an excellent example of how nursing administrators and staff need to change their paradigms to create cost-effective scheduling models.

REFERENCES

Andron, T. M., & Hunter, G. L. (1988). Our experience with a 7-day-on, 7-day-off schedule. *Medical Laboratory Observer, 20,* 42-46.

The demise of the traditional 5-40 workweek? (1981). *American Journal of Nursing, 81,* 1138-1141.

Dison, C. C., Carter, N., & Bromley, P. (1981). Making the change to flex time. *American Journal of Nursing, 81,* 2162-2164.

Donovan, L. (1978). Is there a 7-day work week in your future? *RN, 41*(3), 3-4.

Gowell, Y. M., & Boverie, P. E. (1992). Stress and satisfaction as a result of shift and number of hours worked. *Nursing Administration Quarterly, 16*(4), 14-19.

Gulack, R. (1982). Wanted: Longer (and shorter) shifts . . . plus a little choice in the matter. *RN, 45*(6), 35-39.

Houston, R. (1990). Twelve-hour shifts: Answer to job satisfaction. *Nursing Management, 21*(10), 88f, 88h.

Hutchins, C., & Cleveland, R. (1978). For staff nurses and patients—the 7-70 plan. *American Journal of Nursing, 78,* 230-233.

Larter, M. H. (1982). Creative staffing. In A. Marriner (Ed.), *Contemporary nursing management* (pp. 161-179). St. Louis, MO: C.V. Mosby.

Lillis, Z. (1989). The 12-hour shift: A possible alternative to staffing difficulties. *AARN, 45*(5), 16-17.

O'Connor, L. M. (1994). Event-related sterility assurance. *Surgical Technologist, 26*(1), 8-12.

Rabideau, L., & Skarbek, N. (1978). Our 7-day, 70-hour schedule works. *RN, 41*(3), 5-7.

Schroeter, K. (1994). Implementation of an event-related sterility plan. *AORN Journal, 60,* 595, 598-602.

Slota, M. C., & Balas-Stevens, S. (1990). Implementing and evaluating a change to 12-hour shifts. *Neonatal Network, 8*(6), 51-56.

Stumpf, B. (1989). Staffing and scheduling. In S. Glover (Ed.), *Recruitment and retention* (pp. 72-77). Baltimore: Williams & Wilkins.

Velianoff, G. D. (1991). Establishing a 10-hour schedule. *Nursing Management, 22*(9), 36-38.

Walters, J. A., Puetz, C., Sala, S. M., Hanson, K., Beder, L., Maxson, P., & Crucius, L. (1992). Developing and implementing a tool to measure severity of medication errors. *Journal of Nursing Care Quality, 6*(4), 33-42.

CHAPTER 10

A Managed-Care Methodology for Achieving Cost and Quality Outcomes in Home Health

Virginia L. Maturen

Health care providers, in response to the continuing upward spiral of health care costs, are working to develop delivery systems that provide the appropriate interventions at the appropriate time to achieve the best patient outcomes. This chapter describes a long-term project started by the 10 agency members of VNA *First* to develop a system and the supporting processes to ensure that costly resources are used prudently to achieve maximum consumer benefit and satisfaction. An interdisciplinary group of staff from member agencies recorded their practice for frequently occurring medical diagnoses in a visit-by-visit format to achieve desired patient outcomes. The creation of the critical pathways and resulting patient outcomes (Home Care Steps™ Protocols) has further evolved into a complete clinical documentation system. This system has proven useful to nurse administrators because it offers potential solutions to problems created by both external and internal forces that directly affect overall operations and the delivery of home care services. By analyzing the underlying causes of unachieved outcomes, an agency has data to support its continuous quality improvement program.

VNA *First* is an alliance of 10 Visiting Nurse Associations/ Community Nursing Services serving the northern third of Illinois, eastern Iowa, and northwestern Indiana.[1] In 1991, members of the alliance made a strategic decision to develop Home Care Steps™ Protocols that would position them to respond to changes in the Medicare payment mechanism, namely, Diagnostic Related Groups (DRGs). Although a DRG payment model for home care has not been implemented by the Health Care Financing Administration, other payment models have been introduced to the health care industry, particularly a capitation model defined by an episode of illness (Boling, 1992). The Home Care Steps project combined with a cost/price development model has been found to be equally adaptable for use with several payment mechanisms. While anticipating and positioning themselves for a major change in the payment system, home care agencies have experienced a secondary phenomenon influencing service delivery: An external third party, acting as a "gatekeeper" on behalf of the payer, determines the amount and frequency of home care services a patient will receive.

This set of circumstances led VNA *First* agencies to identify the need for a *practice-based* methodology that was *provider defined* and *internally controlled.* Once they identified these requirements, the development of a provider-controlled managed-care methodology began in earnest. For purposes of this discussion, *managed care* is defined as the "cost containment process in which healthcare benefits are carefully controlled in terms of types, levels, and frequency of treatments; in terms of access to care; and in terms of the amount of reimbursement paid for healthcare services" (Brent, 1991, p. 8; Todd, 1991). In the course of developing the methodology, the group also discovered an important side benefit: By defining practice and predicting outcomes, providers can also begin to measure the quality of their service delivery.

This chapter identifies the components of a proposed methodology for health care service delivery and describes its adaptation to the home care setting. Simultaneously, it describes the features of the process that will enable nurse administrators to predict and control costs better through prudent use of resources while ensuring quality (defined by patient outcomes). The methodology not only addresses issues related to external factors but is helpful in addressing internal challenges that may directly affect operations: variations in individual staff practice patterns, continuity of care, staff shortages, staff retention, documentation of skilled services, and appropriate utilization of all resources.

VNA *First* Home Care Steps are based on the agencies' original work, Home Health CareMaps Tools, and Home Health CoMaps, developed in consultation with the Center for Case Management, Inc., in South Natick, Massachusetts. This initial body of work consisted of developing and field testing Home Health CareMap Tools for 13 high-volume, high-cost medical diagnoses and three complex procedures. Following the successful implementation of its first efforts, VNA *First* member agencies recognized the need for a continued evolution of the project. Now called VNA *First* Home Care Steps Protocols, the managed-care methodology has been further refined and expanded to continue pursuing the goal of positioning the home care industry for health care reform while demonstrating fiscal responsibility and defining quality through outcomes.

UNDERSTANDING THE PROVIDER-CONTROLLED METHODOLOGY

The five components of the provider-controlled Home Care Steps methodology are (a) critical pathways, (b) defined patient outcomes, (c) unit of time, (d) variance identification and tracking, and (e) resource utilization.

Critical Pathways

Critical pathways identify all key interventions or activities for each diagnosis and for each discipline having direct patient contact over the entire episode of illness. These activities or interventions must be correctly timed or sequenced to achieve maximum efficiency and effectiveness of the contact and to achieve a desired set of outcomes. Practitioners involved in direct patient care create the critical pathways and identify the expected outcomes on the basis of their expertise and experience caring for patients with a specific medical diagnosis defined by ICD-9 codes rather than DRGs. The activities and interventions become the standards of practice for each discipline (medicine, nursing, therapies, social work, home care aide, radiology, etc.) but may reflect some local or regional variation in practice. After diagnosis- and discipline-specific practice standards have been identified, the expected outcomes or standards of care can be identified (Goodwin, 1992).

Defined Patient Outcomes

Patient outcomes must be specific, achievable, time limited, and written in measurable language. There must be a mechanism for including the patient, family, and/or caregiver in the process of identifying needs and outcomes unique to the patient and the circumstances (Peters & Eigsti, 1991). Together, the practitioner and the patient, using the Home Care Steps Protocols as a guide, can agree upon an individualized service plan. Then, using the Home Care Steps Protocols for each visit, the practitioner documents the care and teaching given during the course of the visit and the resulting patient reactions and outcomes achieved.

Unit of Time

The time frame is a contact or visit. For home care, this time frame has been clearly defined as a visit. Under a fee-for-service payment system, the visit is also the billable unit. Under an alternative payment mechanism such as a diagnosis-based or capitation model, all patient contacts or visits totaled together equal an episode of care. In anticipation of significant changes in payment for home care and possibly for the entire health care industry, the time frame as defined in the Home Care Steps methodology can be adjusted to specify a billable visit.

Variance Identification and Tracking

When the expected or predicted patient outcomes are not achieved, a variance is said to have occurred. Variances may be either positive or negative. When an outcome is realized more quickly than expected, a positive variance has occurred. When the outcome is not achieved or is achieved more slowly than anticipated, a negative variance has occurred. By analyzing both positive and negative variances, an agency can analyze its strengths and weaknesses and make corrections or enhancements to its own processes and systems. In field testing the Home Care Steps Protocols, VNA *First* member agencies identified four potential sources of variance: (a) patient/caregiver, (b) clinician, (c) system, and (d) community. Some examples of variance from each of these sources are shown in the following chart.

Source	Examples
Patient/caregiver	Cognitive deficit related to problem solving, short-term memory loss, lack of a responsible caregiver
Clinician	Educational and experiential background, critical decision making, individual teaching/communication skills
System	Lack of equipment, untimely referral management
Community	Lack of resources, lack of access to resources

These variance examples can be further subdivided into controllable and uncontrollable variances. It is inevitable that some variance will occur that is beyond an agency's and/or practitioner's scope to control. A patient's loss of memory and the decision by an outside third party to deny payment for extraordinary treatment or services are examples of uncontrollable variances. Examples of controllable variance include late delivery of equipment or the patient's medication not being in the home when the nurse makes the first visit.

It is important for staff to distinguish between controllable and uncontrollable variance so that actions can be taken to ensure that structures and efficient processes are in place to reduce or prevent controllable variance. It may also be possible to change what may be perceived as an uncontrollable variance into a controllable variance. An example is the development of a grant proposal to obtain funding for a van to transport disabled or homebound patients to an adult day care program. Thus an uncontrollable variance, lack of transportation, becomes controllable when patients can be enrolled for the van transport service.

It is likewise important to identify and track uncontrollable variance. Not all patients will achieve all of the expected outcomes 100% of the time, so an agency needs to identify, for a particular patient population, the size and shape of a normal distribution of the outcomes achieved, as well as the size and shape of each standard deviation within the bell-shaped curve. It may be expected that those patients who constitute the negative outliers in a population will use more resources. Such information is essential to an agency's evaluation of their costs for achieving specific quality outcomes and for appropriate pricing to remain competitive. A standardized approach to care based on acceptable practice patterns for a specific disease or condition provides a foundation for collecting, quantifying, and evaluating variance data derived from outcome results.

Resource Utilization

The fifth component in a provider-controlled managed-care methodology is the prediction and tracking of resource utilization. The cost of providing home care services is based on the type and amount of resources utilized to deliver those services. Typically, we think of resources as the staff who have direct patient contact and care responsibilities, such as RNs, physicians, physical and occupational therapists, speech language pathologists, home care workers, and respiratory therapists. But home care may require the utilization of other resources such as durable medical equipment (DME), pharmaceuticals, nutrition supplements, medical and wound care supplies, oxygen, or laboratory services. Tools to predict and track resource utilization by patient and by diagnosis have been developed and are in use by many home care providers. Once resource utilization by case has been identified, costs can be assigned. From this information, the cost per case by diagnosis can be calculated. With the ability to project and track costs, the five components and the supporting tools essential for the development and implementation of a provider-controlled managed-care methodology are complete.

INTEGRATING THE METHODOLOGY
INTO ORGANIZATIONS' DELIVERY SYSTEMS

To meet certification, state licensing, and accreditation requirements, home health agencies must integrate the provider-controlled managed-care methodology into other structures and processes currently in place. Other essential components are clear lines of communication, team meetings, case consultation, and a continuous quality improvement (CQI) program.

Communication is essential to the overall coordination of services. Practitioners providing direct patient care must discuss service plans and patient responses with all other members of the agency's multidisciplinary team. Similarly, if two or more RNs provide visits to a patient or there is use of temporary or relief staff to complement the agency's own employees, staff of the same discipline must communicate visit plans and outcome results to ensure efficiency and continuity of care. Communication must occur with practitioners at other points in the health care system, the patient's primary physician, case managers and third-party payers, direct care personnel in the acute hospital, the skilled nursing facility, the adult day care center, the DME provider, and so forth. Finally, all direct caregivers must communicate with the patient and family members and actively involve them in their own health care recovery.

Team meetings and interdisciplinary team conferences give staff a regular setting in which to evaluate patient progress in terms of outcome achievement. If outcomes are not achieved, the type and frequency of variance occurrence must be tabulated and analyzed so that appropriate adjustments in the service plan can be made. The frequent occurrence of variance may signal the need for additional involvement of resources such as consultation with the medical social worker or mental health clinical specialist. In making the decision to use additional resources, agency policy may require review and refinement, especially when uncontrollable variances contribute to the patient's short-term and long-term service needs. In a provider-controlled managed-care system, policies related to decisions about increasing or decreasing services in response to variance events must be clearly stated.

When individual patient variances occur, there should be mechanisms in place to evaluate the underlying causes of the controllable variances. The tools and the analysis should be individualized to the agency and possibly further, to the program or operations levels. Examining causes of variance provides information for continuous quality improvement. For example, the variance category *lack of equipment* may be further examined by tracking additional subcategories such as (a) late delivery, (b) equipment malfunction, (c) equipment not available from supplier, (d) payer will not authorize payment, (e) patient unable to purchase, and (f) order received late and not filled. By further detailing and examining the variance etiology, corrections or adjustments in the systems can be made to prevent further occurrences related to some causes.

OVERCOMING BARRIERS TO THE ADAPTATION OF THE METHODOLOGY TO HOME CARE

Barriers to adapting and implementing a managed-care methodology in the home care setting include selecting the diagnoses, defining the time element and service goals, streamlining the paperwork, individualizing the protocols for each patient, addressing the needs of patients with multiple diagnoses, and tailoring the protocols to the agency's individual needs.

Selecting the Diagnoses

During the course of developing the project, adapting the methodology to home care, and gaining member consensus, many issues were identified and discussed. In selecting the ICD-9 codes, referral and admitting diagnoses from all member agencies were tabulated to ensure the selection of the high-volume, high-cost diagnoses. However, in selecting the high-volume diagnoses, a certain amount of risk was assumed because patient populations with these diagnoses are affected by many variables and pose an increased risk for inaccuracies in predicting outcome achievement.

Defining the Time Element and Service Goals

The time element was and still is defined as a visit because the visit remains the billable unit under a fee-for-visit payment mechanism. Attempts to define the time element as a week or a module proved unsuccessful and were discarded.

Overall service goals can be categorized into several general headings: activities of daily living (ADL) function, medication management, knowledge of disease process and disease management, transfers and ambulation, prevention of complications, caregiver support, symptom control, and discharge status (Lalonde, 1988). Categorizing goals provided a guide for developing diagnosis- and visit-specific outcomes directly linked to the interventions defined for every visit. Breaking the goals into several derivative outcomes allows for more precision and accuracy when quantifying and qualifying patient progress along a continuum.

Streamlining the Paperwork

The work of defining practice and its associated outcomes required the development of a format to support the use of the protocols for documentation. The format has undergone significant changes to create tools that can be used by all disciplines for documentation of the skilled visit. Although the documentation capabilities, as presented, may not reduce documentation time per se (the basic requirements by the regulating bodies have not changed), streamlining the system to allow checks and zeros to indicate activities and outcomes achieved or not achieved resulted in more thorough and comprehensive documentation.

Individualizing the Protocols for Each Patient

Throughout the discussions and field testing, the need for individualization of the protocols remained foremost in the minds of the creators. Consequently there are ample provisions for the individualization of all the diagnosis-specific Home Care Steps Protocols. For example, patient assessment parameters, long-term goals, the use of teaching tools, and visit frequencies must all be tailored to the needs of each patient and family. Each patient possesses his or her own unique circumstances and learning needs. Any standardized practice patterns must be fine-tuned to the patient's needs and unique set of responses.

Managing Patients With Multiple Diagnoses

A major issue requiring continued thought and work has been the dilemma posed by patients with multiple diagnoses and/or history of chronic disease. Additional conditions related to a patient's primary diagnosis introduce additional variables into an already less than predictable situation. VNA *First*'s member agencies embrace a philosophical approach of holistic patient and family care. The need to address other actual or potential problems during the course of service delivery was viewed as essential to the successful delineation of the methodology components and eventual implementation of the project. The result was the development of the Home CoSteps as a derivative tool of the Home Care Steps Protocols. The CoSteps define desired outcomes for each additional diagnosis or problem presented and may be used separately or integrated into the skilled-visit report note.

At present, project members do not believe that they have yet found a satisfactory solution to the dilemma of managing the care of patients with long-term chronic illnesses or handicaps or patients described as "frail elderly." The group continues to seek other alternatives that may be used in combination with the delivery system as it has evolved.

Tailoring the Protocols to
Meet Agencies' Individual Needs

Field testing itself created some problems in that all participating agencies defined their own unique set of policies and procedures related to the activity of documentation. Therefore project team members agreed that using the protocols for documentation versus using them as a guide to care had to be determined by each agency. Furthermore, decisions related to individual patient requirements, and thus some interpretation of how and when to use protocols and which of the protocols to use, would also have to be taken into consideration.

With the Home Care Steps Protocols for Documentation and Staff Guidance, VNA *First*'s Home Care Steps Protocols were designed for use (a) as a clinical documentation system and (b) as a guide for new staff and relief (temporary) staff for planning and delivering care. The design has purposely been kept flexible to be integrated easily with portions of an agency's existing system and to allow for minimal modifications to reflect regional differences in treatment and practice patterns. The work is continually reviewed to ensure compliance with regulatory, licensing, and accreditation requirements.

The clinical documentation system contains seven components: (a) admission visit note, (b) diagnosis-specific fact sheet (see Figure 10.1), (c) diagnosis/visit-specific note (see Figure 10.2), (d) clinical assessment form, (e) narrative addendum, (f) discharge visit note, and (g) discharge summary note.

All disciplines can use the same format for documentation, but content will vary because it is both diagnosis- and discipline-specific for every visit. Components 1, 2, 3, and 6 contain the field-tested critical pathways and patient outcomes. Agencies may substitute their own forms for the remaining components.

This clinical documentation system works best when the staff have access to patient information and visit-specific outcome achievement. This access may be achieved through daily office visits to review patient records, a traveling chart system, or a home chart option. Tracking patient outcome achievement via the paper-based system is difficult at best. A mechanism to ensure routine access to the patient's clinical record increases successful tracking of outcomes and follow-up on variances.

The protocols provide a comprehensive guide for new staff, temporary staff, and experienced staff. Because the protocols list all the care and instructional activities related to a specific diagnosis, they also serve as a communication tool that promotes continuity of care among all staff and all disciplines involved with the patient.

As previously discussed, project members felt strongly about the need to identify a mechanism that would guide the care and instruction needed by a

CONGESTIVE HEART FAILURE *HOME CARE STEPS*™

Patient Name: _____

ID#: _____

Date *Home Care Steps*™ protocols Opened:_____ Closed: _____ Start of Care:_____

ASSESS/OBSERVE: (Choose appropriate ones)   OTHER *Home Care Steps*™ or Care Plans:

___ Cardiovascular Assessment/Vital Signs
___ Weight
___ Lung Sounds
___ Assess for: ___ fatigue   ___ orthopnea
                  ___ dyspnea   ___ anorexia
                  ___ cough   ___ mobility
                  ___ edema   ___ emotional status
___ Other: _____

NURSING DIAGNOSES: (Choose appropriate diagnoses)

___ 1. Knowledge deficit regarding disease process and home care management.
___ 2. Alteration in cardiac output related to mechanical factors.
___ 3. Alteration in fluid volume; excess, related to increased systemic venous congestion and/or right ventricular failure.
___ 4. Potential for alteration in skin integrity related to edema.
___ 5. Ineffective coping related to diagnosis and prognosis.
___ Other: _____

LONG TERM GOALS:

1. Patient/caregiver will demonstrate understanding of disease process and self-care management.
2. Patient will have improved cardiac output.
3. Patient will have a more stable fluid balance.
4. Patient will have intact skin surface (or absence of signs and symptoms of infection from skin breakdown).
5. Patient's vital signs, weight and cardiovascular status are normal for patient range.
Other: _____

TEACHING TOOLS: **VARIANCE CODES:**
_____   V1 - Patient too sick   V5 - Lack of Equipment
_____   V2 - Co-Morbid Interference   V6 - Patient or Caregiver Decision
_____   V3 - Patient's Cognitive Status V7 - Other (explain)
_____   V4 - Lack of Caregiver   V8 - Not Applicable (explain)

SN VISIT FREQUENCY:

Recommended: 3 wk x 2, 2 wk x 3, 1 wk x 4   Ordered: _____
                  (16 visits total)

Other Disciplines: _____

_____
Signature and Title

Home Care Steps protocols are designed to address the patient's acute episode of illness. Visit intensity and frequency may also be influenced by the patient's unique set of circumstances, including but not limited to the home environment, resources, presence of life-supporting therapies, and the presence of other chronic illnesses or limiting handicaps.

Figure 10.1. Congestive Heart Failure Home Care Steps
SOURCE: VNA *First.*

patient with a secondary or unrelated diagnosis. To address the needs of patients with a history of chronic disease or multiple diagnoses, the task force

CHF *Home Care Steps*™   Patient Name:_____ ID#:_____
Visit 2   Date:_____

Care Elements	Interventions: Use "✓" for complete; "0" for not done.	Comments
DISEASE PROCESS	Instruct patient regarding signs and symptoms of CHF.___	
MEDICATION	Review medication schedule.___ Instruct purpose, action, side effects of following medication(s): _____ _____ _____ Set up medi-planner if appropriate.___	
NUTRITION/ HYDRATION	Assess prior knowledge regarding dietary and fluid restrictions.___ Instruct regarding fluid restrictions___ and basic low sodium restrictions.___	
ACTIVITY	Instruct to avoid over-exertion; frequent rest periods.___	
SAFETY	Reassess for environmental hazards, including oxygen and modify as appropriate.___ Assess understanding of how and when to call for help.___	
TREATMENTS	Weigh patient (on patient's own scale, if available).___ Check vital signs.___ Assess for shortness of breath.___ edema.___ Review use of oxygen (if ordered) and oxygen precautions.___	
TESTS	As ordered._____	
PSYCHO/ SOCIAL	Assess patient/caregiver coping skills/learning ability.___	
INTERTEAM SERVICES/ COMMUNITY REFERRALS	Assess ability to purchase necessary supplies, food, etc., for treatment.___ Assess need for additional community resources.___ Case conference: __MSW, __PT, __OT, __SLP, __HHA, __MD, __Other.___ Next MD appointment (date)._____ Review plan of care for home care services.___	

Patient Outcomes	Met	Not Met	Explain Variance Code Identified in *Not Met* Column
1. States signs and symptoms of CHF.			
2. Verbalizes purpose, action, side effects of each medication instructed (as listed above).			
3. States how and when to call for help.			
4. Verbalizes basic home safety precautions.			
5. Verbalizes need to avoid exertion and to rest frequently.			
6. Verbalizes general diet/fluid restrictions.			
7. Verbalizes and agrees to plan of care for services.			

PLAN FOR NEXT VISIT: _____
_____

PHYSICIAN CONTACT: _____

OUTCOME OF MD CONTACT: _____
_____

Signature and Title

Figure 10.2. CHF Home Care Steps Visit 2
SOURCE: VNA *First.*

members developed one further component, the companion system of CoSteps (see Figure 10.3). Each CoStep tool consists of two components:

HYPERTENSION *CoStep*

Patient Name: _____

This diagnosis is: _____ new   ID#: _____
                   _____ exacerbation
                   _____ chronic condition   Start of Care: _____

GOALS					
Verbalizes and/or demonstrates knowledge and behavior necessary to manage disease.					
PATIENT OUTCOMES Dates:					
1.	Verbalizes three (3) signs and symptoms to be reported to RN/MD.					
2.	Verbalizes importance of compliance with medication schedule.					
3.	Verbalizes importance of slow position change.					
4.	Verbalizes sources of hidden sodium in commercial foods.					
5.	Verbalizes two (2) measures to reduce stress.					
6.	Identifies and explains "at risk" behaviors to alter.					
7.	Explains the disease process and treatment principles.					
8.	Other:					
	Initials:					

RN Signatures:

Outcome Codes

M = Met   _____
NM = Not Met   _____
                           _____

Home Care Steps™   Copyright© 1994, VNA First, All Rights Reserved

Figure 10.3. Hypertension CoStep
SOURCE: VNA *First.*

1. Goal(s): Long-term goal(s) focusing on the continued management of a stable diagnosis or condition.

2. Patient Outcomes: Appropriate outcomes (listed in priority order) required for the patient to continue the independent management of any secondary diagnoses. When the nurse verifies that the patient has met the outcomes, a dated note should be made.

Like the Home Care Steps Protocols, the CoSteps may be used as a guide or integrated into the clinical documentation system. Using the companion CoStep system allows optimal flexibility and individualization of patient care, with the care and teaching content appropriately dispersed over the episode of care to prevent overwhelming the patient with too much information. The tools allow for improved efficiency of visits with the earliest possible discharge of the patient according to his or her abilities and documented achievement of outcomes.

EVALUATING VARIANCE DATA

The data that result from the identification and tracking of variance, described earlier in this chapter, provide valuable information about an agency's strengths and weaknesses. To assist with the analysis of variance data resulting from the use of the Home Care Steps Protocols, three tools have been developed for data collection:

1. *Overview of Variance Occurrence:* Provides a matrix that allows for the identification of variances by diagnosis.
2. *Variance Close-Up:* Tracks variance data by individual patient and by specific diagnosis and documents actual outcome achievement for *each* visit.
3. *Patient Outcome Summary:* Identifies actual outcome achievement for the individual patient. It allows for the immediate assessment of the patient's progress or lack of progress.

Refinement of each of these tools and the examination of detailed data should be individualized at the agency level. Through careful analysis of variance causation, an agency will be able to identify weaknesses or strengths in their processes or systems and make needed modifications or build strengths.

PREDICTING AND TRACKING
RESOURCE UTILIZATION

Although the Home Care Steps Protocols are designed to predict clinical outcomes, the next logical step is to identify resource utilization and assign costs. In addition to identifying the staff resources used to make direct patient contact or complete a home visit, the critical pathways can identify all the other resources required to support the patient at home. For example, if a patient is receiving intravenous (IV) antibiotics at home, then the cost of the medication, supplies, pump, IV pole, equipment delivery, and laboratory services becomes significant. If the patient has a resolving lung condition, home x-ray and oxygen support may be an added cost. Standardized tools can be designed to predict costs, identify actual costs, and identify the total cost per diagnosis, per episode of illness.

FUTURE DIRECTIONS

Despite the difficulties of developing a provider-controlled managed-care methodology, early studies by VNA *First*'s member agencies have identified many advantages in its use. Staff reported enhanced understanding of home care services, improved time management, improved documentation, and increased continuity of patient care. Managers identified benefits such as "equalization" of staff regardless of education and experience; improved coordination and continuity of care; improved assessment of staff education needs, patient teaching needs, and support materials; and improved consistency with policies and procedures. Administrators reported using the data generated by the methodology to support agency CQI programs and accreditation reviews, improve projection and tracking of resource utilization, and facilitate program development and marketing.

As this project continues, user group members have identified an urgent need to automate the Home Care Steps Protocols, together with the clinical documentation, variance tracking, and resource utilization tools. New Home Care Steps Protocols are needed for additional acute diagnoses, chronic disease, and long-term care needs of patients. Some existing protocols may be further fine-tuned to correspond with patient acuity levels. Finally, the provider-controlled managed-care methodology needs integration with other providers and systems across the health care continuum as we move toward a national health care policy.

CONCLUSION

Nurse administrators are increasingly being called upon to demonstrate to payers and consumers both fiscal and ethical accountability for delivering appropriate care at the appropriate time while achieving the best patient outcomes. The Home Care Steps Protocols described in this chapter offer nurse administrators in home health care the process and the tools to meet these demands. Though originally developed to respond to changes in payment mechanisms, the protocols have evolved into a complete clinical documentation system that serves multiple functions. In addition to documenting the nursing interventions and patient outcomes, the protocols provide data that can be used to improve continuity of care, continuing quality improvement efforts, staff orientation and development, service projection, and budgeting.

For the nurse administrator in any setting, the concept of a provider-controlled managed-care methodology addresses the need for cost control while placing the primary focus where it belongs, on the patient and the outcomes of care.

NOTE

1. The 10 member agencies of VNA *First* are Community Nursing Service of DuPage, and Community Nursing Service West, Oak Park, Illinois; Visiting Nurse Association of Chicago; Visiting Nurse Association of Fox Valley, Aurora, Illinois; Visiting Nurse Association North, Skokie, Illinois; Visiting Nurse Association NW Indiana; Visiting Nurse Association of the Rockford Area; Genesis Visiting Nurse Association (Davenport, Iowa); Visiting Nurse and Homemaker Association of Rock Island County, and West Towns Visiting Nursing Service, Berwyn, Illinois.

REFERENCES

Boling, J. (1992). An American integrated health care system? Where are we now? *Case Manager,* *3*(3), 53-59.

Brent, N. (1991). Managed care: Legal and ethical implications. *Home Health Care Nurse, 9*(3), 8-10.

Goodwin, D. (1992). Critical pathways in home health care. *Journal of Nursing Administration,* *22*(2), 35-40.

Lalonde, B. (1988). Assuring the quality of home care via the assessment of client outcomes. *Caring,* *12*(1), 20-24.

Peters, D., & Eigsti, D. (1991). Utilizing outcomes in home care. *Caring, 10*(10), 44-51.

Todd, K. M. (1991). Managed care. *CDS Review, 9*(3).

Practice-Based Evaluation
of Outcomes Management

Part 3 is a logical capstone to a volume dedicated to outcomes of effective management practices. The contributed chapters describe a variety of practice-based evaluation research projects throughout North America.

Mitchell-DiCenso, Pinelli, and Southwell (Chapter 11) describe the assessment of need, implementation of roles, and evaluation of outcomes for a project that expanded advance-practice nursing roles in an Ontario, Canada, neonatology unit. Outcomes were measured in terms of safety, efficacy, quality of care, patient satisfaction, costs, provider job satisfaction, autonomy, and quality of work life.

Case management on a rehabilitation unit is the setting for Chapter 12, by Wells, Holder, and Dengler. They report on a pilot project in which process and outcomes of a nurse-managed, multidisciplinary clinical pathway were tested. Outcomes measured include patient outcomes of goal attainment, length of stay, charges, and satisfaction of staff.

In Chapter 13, Sebastian, Hagan, Bayer, McNamara, and Combs describe program evaluation in long-term care, comparing methods used to evaluate care in institutional and noninstitutional units providing care to frail elderly clients. The goals of care on these units serving similar client populations drove the evaluation methods as well as the outcomes measures appropriate to measure goal achievement.

A research-based project provided the framework for Chapter 14, by Blegen and Murphy. This study of a sample of women having elective cesarean section focuses on outcomes of resource use and clinical status and provides important insights into successful cost analysis of an innovation.

The final chapter of Part 3 addresses an ongoing concern of many health care managers in this decade: evaluating a redesign program. Stetler, Creer, and Effken describe an effort designed to evaluate the effectiveness of a broad-based redesign program. They discuss a utilization-focused program evaluation, formative and summative evaluation implementation, and the factors that can influence outcomes at every state of evaluation.

Like the other parts and chapters, Part 3 has been designed to provoke critical thinking and the reader's expansion of the concepts and the work shared by the contributing authors.

CHAPTER 11

Introduction and Evaluation of an Advanced Nursing Practice Role in Neonatal Intensive Care

Alba Mitchell-DiCenso
Janet Pinelli
Doris Southwell

Efforts by the government of the province of Ontario to reduce the number of physicians and by the nursing profession to develop advanced nursing practice roles afforded an opportunity to develop an expanded role for nurses in neonatology. We have used research methods to assess the need for clinical nurse specialist/neonatal practitioners (CNS/NPs) in tertiary-level neonatal intensive care units (NICUs); to define the CNS/NP role; to determine the educational preparation required for the role; to evaluate the educational program in terms of knowledge and problem-solving, communication, and clinical skills; to evaluate the role in terms of safety, efficacy, quality of care, parent satisfaction, and costs; to assess the job satisfaction of CNS/NPs working in the role for at least 1 year; and to evaluate the impact of CNS/NPs on the job satisfaction, autonomy, and quality of work life of other members of the health care team.

The search for more cost-effective strategies to deliver health care and the nursing profession's emphasis on the development of advanced nursing roles have afforded the opportunity to consider expanded roles for nurses in a variety of health care settings. A major change in the delivery of health services should be based on scientific evidence where possible. In this chapter, we outline a framework that we used to introduce and evaluate an expanded role for nurses in tertiary-level neonatal intensive care units (NICUs) in Ontario, Canada. The framework that guided our work may be useful to nursing administrators who are faced with the challenge of introducing advanced nursing roles in primary, secondary, or tertiary health care settings.

FRAMEWORK FOR INTRODUCING
NEW ROLES FOR HEALTH PROFESSIONALS

We adapted an existing framework (Spitzer, 1978) for introducing new roles for health professionals to encompass 10 steps (Table 11.1). Each step of the framework will be described, followed by a description of our activities specific to the neonatal advanced-practice nursing role.

Step 1: Is There a Need for the
New Approach to Patient Care?

First, it is important to establish or verify the actual need for the new role. This requires the examination of developments in health care delivery in terms of changes in the quantity, distribution, or roles of health care personnel traditionally providing the care and in terms of changes in patient numbers or acuity. The need for a new approach to patient care may be substantiated if the supply of health care personnel is inadequate to meet the demand for health care services.

Valid surveys are an irreplaceable prelude to the introduction of major changes in a health provider's role (Spitzer, 1978). To determine whether an imbalance existed between the supply of physicians and the demand for medical services in tertiary-level NICUs in Ontario, Canada, the medical directors, head nurses, and staff physicians of the nine tertiary-level NICUs in Ontario and the directors of the five postgraduate pediatric residency programs were surveyed. To evaluate the supply of physicians, data were collected about the numbers of physicians, including residents, staffing the units each shift over the past 5 years, and the percentage of time spent in direct patient care. To evaluate the demand for medical services, annual data for the previous 5 years were collected, including number of admissions to the NICU according to birthweight, length of stay, ventilator patient-days, patient acuity, rates of transfer out of the NICU, and occupancy rates.

On the basis of the information gathered from these surveys, it was concluded that there was a disequilibrium in the NICUs because workload exceeded the availability of medical staff (Paes et al., 1989). Given the political emphasis on reducing the number of residency positions, it was clear that the increased need for health care services would have to be met by alternatives to

TABLE 11.1 Framework for Introducing and Evaluating New Roles for
Health Professionals

1. Is there a need for the new approach to patient care?

2. What is the definition of the new role?

3. What educational preparation is required to assume the new role?

4. Is the new approach to patient care safe and effective?

5. Does the introduction of the new role affect the quality of care rendered?

6. What is the acceptance and satisfaction level of those receiving care from the new health professional?

7. Is the new approach to patient care economically efficient?

8. What are the satisfaction levels of all health professionals affected directly or indirectly by the new approach to patient care?

9. Has a transfer of function occurred from the health professional traditionally performing the role to the new health professional?

10. Has long-term surveillance been conducted to monitor change over time in performance and change in provider and client attitude toward the role?

physicians such as physician assistants, respiratory therapists, or nurse practitioners. Examination of these alternatives by leaders of the nursing professional organizations, academic physicians, the provincial ministry of health, and NICU nursing and medical administrators revealed strong support for the nurse practitioner. The group opposed the inclusion of physician assistants because this would add another member to the health care team with the potential for fragmenting patient care. They opposed respiratory therapists because their role would be more narrowly defined than that of the nurse practitioner.

Step 2: What Is the Definition of the New Role?

Once the need for the new role is determined, it is important to define, as precisely as possible, what the new role will entail. Because of the potential controversy that the introduction of a new role can create, it is important to gather data from key individuals.

To define the role of the nurse practitioner in the NICU, we surveyed medical directors, head nurses, directors of nursing, staff nurses, and staff physicians in Ontario tertiary-level NICUs. In addition, we surveyed a random sample of certified neonatal nurse practitioners (NNPs) in 40 U.S. states and one Canadian province and a convenience sample of medical directors and head nurses of NICUs in 20 U.S. states and one Canadian province that employ NNPs. To learn about the existing NP role, we visited NICUs in three U.S. cities and one hospital in Canada that employed NNPs. On the basis of survey responses, the role was defined to include clinical, educational, research, and administrative responsibilities, with the majority of time (70-75%) allocated to clinical practice. Given the breadth of this role and the advanced clinical practice, these individuals were given the title of *clinical nurse specialist/neonatal practitioner* (CNS/NP). This title reflects the merging of the traditional roles of the CNS and NP, as described in the literature (Elder & Bullough, 1990; Kitzman, 1989). Because of the diversity of types of NP programs and the range of practice levels that exists, it was felt that the singular term *NP* might be interpreted as a physician replacement for technical skill performance rather than as a professional nurse in an advanced nursing practice role. Because a traditional CNS clinical practice role may not necessarily combine skills in patient management with expertise in clinical assessment and diagnosis, the *nurse practitioner* designation was added to the title.

Clinically, the CNS/NP assumes primary responsibility for transporting outborn neonates or attending the delivery, obtaining a thorough maternal history and documenting pertinent findings relative to the infant's presentation at birth, assessing the physical and developmental status of the infant, identifying primary and secondary medical problems, developing and implementing a plan for the management of each problem, revising management plans upon periodic reassessment of the infant's problems, and developing discharge plans. At daily rounds, the CNS/NP discusses assessment and management plans with the attending neonatologist. The CNS/NP then carries out the diagnostic and treatment regimen without further consultation. When unusual or unexpected changes in the neonate's status develop that require an alteration in management, the CNS/NP consults with the neonatologist to reevaluate the neonate's status and to decide upon further management. Approval for CNS/NPs to perform specific delegated medical acts was obtained through the College of Physicians and Surgeons of Ontario.

In their educational role, CNS/NPs share responsibility for teaching rounds and conferences and participate in the clinical education of nursing students, residents, staff nurses, and parents of infants. Their research participation includes the critical appraisal of research data and implementation of findings in patient care decisions, the identification of areas in which research is required, and participation on research teams. Administrative activities include participation on selected committees and in quality care review (Hunsberger et al., 1992).

CNS/NPs are hired through a collaborative process involving the director of nursing, the NICU head nurse, and the NICU medical director. They are accountable to the medical director for delegated medical responsibilities and to the director of nursing for other aspects of their role. They are evaluated jointly by the director of nursing and the NICU medical director with input from the head nurse and peers and by self-assessment.

Step 3: What Educational Preparation
Is Required to Assume the New Role?

Once the new role is delineated, it is important to develop an educational program to prepare individuals to perform the role competently.

To determine the educational preparation required for the CNS/NPs, nurse educators in every NNP graduate program in the United States were surveyed to learn about admission criteria, program objectives, length of program, and range of content included. In addition, nurse educators from NNP educational programs located in three cities in the United States were consulted (Hunsberger et al., 1992).

On the basis of the data collected, it was decided to prepare these individuals at the graduate level. A neonatal stream was integrated into the existing Master of Health Sciences program at McMaster University. This is a 16-month educational program that includes 600 didactic hours and over 700 hours of supervised clinical practice.

An essential component of an appraisal of the new role is an evaluation of the educational program in which the health professional was prepared (Spitzer, 1978). Two evaluations of the educational program have been completed: One found that graduating CNS/NPs scored higher than first year CNS/NP students in knowledge and problem solving (Mitchell, Watts, et al., 1995), and another found that graduating CNS/NPs had scores equivalent to those of second-year pediatric residents in knowledge and in problem-solving, communication, and clinical skills (Mitchell et al., 1991).

Step 4: Is the New Approach to
Patient Care Safe and Effective?

Spitzer (1978) explained that before new professionals become permanently assimilated into the present health care system, their performance should stand the same rigorous scrutiny as any major new therapy or drug.

To determine the safety and effectiveness of the CNS/NPs, the first randomized controlled trial to evaluate neonatal nurse practitioners was conducted (Mitchell, Guyatt, Marrin, et al., in press). A randomized controlled trial is the most rigorous design to evaluate an intervention—in this case, the substitution of care providers—because it minimizes study biases and ensures that the experimental and control groups are similar in all aspects except the intervention of interest.

All 821 infants admitted to the NICU at McMaster Division of Chedoke-McMaster Hospitals in Hamilton, Ontario, between September 16, 1991, and September 15, 1992, were randomized to care by a CNS/NP team or to care by a pediatric resident team. The CNS/NP team included CNS/NPs who provided care to 414 neonates during the day and pediatric residents who provided care to the neonates from 1600 to 0800 hours. The pediatric resident team included pediatric residents who provided round-the-clock care for 407 neonates. Each team was supervised by one neonatal fellow and one neonatologist. One might view this evaluation as limited because the CNS/NPs provided care only during the day, with overnight coverage provided by the residents. Most NICUs provide far less intense coverage during the night than the day, and those covering at night generally respond to changes in patient status or emergencies only, rather than taking part in the comprehensive planning of care that occurs during the day. Given that the majority of management decisions regarding the care of the neonate are made during the day and given that most NICUs do not employ enough CNS/NPs to provide 24-hour coverage 7 days a week, medical directors of NICUs have preferred this staffing arrangement.

There were no statistically significant differences between the CNS/NP team and the resident team in number of neonate deaths and in infant morbidity as measured by the Neonatal Health Index (Scott, Bauer, Kraemer, & Tyson, 1989), and by number of neonates experiencing complications resulting from incorrect medical management decisions. Both teams also scored similarly in the measurement of long-term outcomes at 8 months of age, adjusted for prematurity, using the Minnesota Infant Development Inventory (Creighton & Sauve, 1988). The manuscript describing this trial in detail is soon to be published by *Pediatrics* (Mitchell, Guyatt, Marrin, et al., in press).

Step 5: Does the Introduction of the New Role Affect the Quality of Care Rendered?

In addition to assessment of safety and efficacy by assessing health outcomes, it also is important to determine whether the introduction of the new role affects the quality of care rendered (Spitzer, 1978). The assessment of quality of care permits evaluation of the process of care rather than outcome of care. Given that some outcomes are determined by factors other than the quality of care provided, it is unfair to fault a clinician if the patient's condition deteriorates. Therefore process measures evaluate the quality of the care provider's actions: for example, investigation orders, drug prescriptions, and patient education.

One approach to the evaluation of quality of care is through the use of indicator conditions. Indicator conditions are distinct clinical entities such as symptoms, disease states, complications, or injuries that occur frequently in the type of practice under surveillance and in which the outcome can be affected favorably or adversely by the choice of treatment. This technique, introduced by Kessner, Kalk, and Singer (1973) and refined by Sibley et al. (1975), has been shown to be a valid and practical measure of quality of care (Buhler, Glick, & Sheps, 1988; Chambers, Sibley, Spitzer, & Tugwell, 1981; Sheps & Robertson, 1984; Sibley et al., 1975). Through review of charts of all neonates in the randomized controlled trial, the quality of care provided by the CNS/NP team was compared with that provided by the resident team by evaluating the management of 14 specifically designed indicator conditions. The adequacy of management for the indicator conditions was rated according to explicit criteria that had been established by a professional peer group of neonatologists and that had been tested for validity and reliability (Marrin, Paes, Mitchell, & Southwell, 1993). In only two instances did differences between the two groups achieve statistical significance. These were in the assessment and management of jaundice and in charting. The CNS/NP team did better in meeting criteria for both these indicator conditions, though in both cases the differences between the groups were small and unlikely to be clinically important.

Step 6: What Is the Acceptance and Satisfaction Level of Those Receiving Care From the New Health Professional?

It is important that consumers willingly accept care from the health providers in the new role and that consumers be satisfied with the care they receive (Spitzer, 1978).

Parents' satisfaction with the medical care provided to their infant was measured in the randomized controlled trial by a specially designed Neonatal Instrument of Parent Satisfaction With Care (NIPS) that had established reliability and validity (Mitchell, Guyatt, Paes, et al., in press). There were no statistically significant differences between the two groups in terms of parent satisfaction.

Step 7: Is the New Approach to Patient Care Economically Efficient?

The evaluation of the economic impact of the new method of health care delivery from the standpoint of society and government is most important (Spitzer, 1978). However, the measurement of the cost-effectiveness of any new health care provider is highly complex because of the number of factors that should be measured. These include productivity, or the number of patients cared for; reimbursement method, source, and amount; training costs; use of resources—for example, diagnostic tests; and whether those who traditionally performed the role fill the freed-up time with other income-driven services.

In the randomized controlled trial, data were collected on salaries of all health care providers included in the care of the neonates, costs of every medical service provided to each infant, and family expenses incurred while the infant was in the NICU. There were no statistically significant differences in the costs of care provided by the two teams.

Step 8: What Are the Satisfaction Levels of All Health Professionals Affected Directly or Indirectly by the New Approach to Patient Care?

As part of the overall evaluation that accompanies the introduction of a new role for health providers, satisfaction levels of all health professionals affected directly or indirectly by the change need to be assessed. Without such information, serious errors about the feasibility of widespread implementation of the new role can be made (Spitzer, 1978).

Each year since CNS/NPs were introduced into the NICUs, they have been surveyed regarding their role and their satisfaction with the role. Consistently, they report a high degree of satisfaction with their role. All 16 CNS/NPs working in the role for at least 1 year in 1994 responded to the survey and noted the positive aspects of the role as the autonomy it provides, the diverse nature of the role, access to knowledge, the variety of challenging clinical experiences, the opportunity to provide holistic care, caring for infants from birth to discharge, being able to support and educate staff nurses, feeling like valued members of a multidisciplinary health care team, working with CNS/NP colleagues, and having flexibility in scheduling and activities. Negative aspects of the role included insufficient financial compensation, being too busy, the political struggle between medicine and nursing, and the heavy clinical component without enough time for research. Those working alone in their setting reported a lack of support.

The impact of the nurse practitioner role on all NICU caregivers was examined in terms of job satisfaction, autonomy, quality of life, and clinical decision making. Eighty-eight percent of all caregivers said the CNS/NP made a difference to their level of satisfaction. Of these caregivers, 46% reported no change in their autonomy and 44% reported increased autonomy since the CNS/NP was introduced into the NICU. All respiratory therapists reported that CNS/NP presence in the NICU had diminished their quality of life, whereas the other caregivers reported improvement (86%) or no change (14%). If given a choice, 96% of the staff nurses preferred to work on a team with a CNS/NP compared with a team with a resident. Respondents reported that CNS/NPs provide a collaborative atmosphere, are good sources of information, assume leadership and decision-making roles in their practice, and provide consistent care of patients and families. Crowding in working areas when there are too many trainees at the bedside was listed among the negative aspects of working in a NICU that employs CNS/NPs.

Step 9: Has a Transfer of Function Occurred From the Health Professional Traditionally Performing the Role to the New Health Professional?

It is essential to determine whether the objectives about changes in role and about behavioral characteristics of new health professionals have been met in actual practice (Spitzer, 1978). Before, during, and since the completion of the randomized controlled trial, the CNS/NP team has managed the care of half of the admissions into the NICU, and the other half has been managed by the pediatric resident team. The expectations of both teams for patient care and for accountability to the supervising neonatologist are the same. All members of the health care team, including consultants, pharmacists, social workers, and respiratory therapists, relate to the CNS/NPs as providers with primary responsibility for the health care management of the neonate rather than in the original staff nurse role they performed.

Step 10: Has Long-Term Surveillance Been Conducted to Monitor Change Over Time in Performance and Change in Provider and Client Attitude Toward the Role?

Long-term follow-up of the new role is essential in identifying any shifts that might cause concern years after the role is implemented. There may be a change in the public attitude toward the new role, especially in areas in which physician shortages can be corrected. Those in the new role may experience dissatisfaction or burnout, and it may become difficult to recruit new candidates for the role. Negative incidents such as preventable deaths, avoidable harm to patients, and lawsuits could occur in patterns or with a frequency that would force second thoughts about the whole concept (Spitzer, 1978).

Ongoing surveillance of the CNS/NP role to detect problems or benefits over the long term is occurring through annual surveys of the CNS/NPs and through regular meetings of an advisory committee that includes a CNS/NP, the director of nursing, the coordinator of the CNS/NP educational program, the director of the School of Nursing, the medical director of the NICU, the chair of the Department of Pediatrics, the director of the postgraduate pediatric residency program, and a neonatologist.

ISSUES RELATED TO THE INTRODUCTION
AND EVALUATION OF CNS/NPs

The process of introducing and evaluating CNS/NPs in tertiary-level NICUs posed a number of contentious issues that had to be addressed. These issues are described below.

Support for the Role

The successful introduction of a new role for a health care provider requires the support of key individuals. For this reason, the first activity undertaken when considering the introduction of CNS/NPs into NICUs in Ontario was the formation of the advisory committee described above. Every decision made regarding the need for CNS/NPs, their role, their educational preparation, and their evaluation was vetted by this committee, which included nursing and physician educators, clinicians, researchers, and administrators. Numerous contentious issues were discussed at length by this committee, but once these were resolved, each member was able to defend the decisions with his or her respective colleagues within and outside his or her own institution and with government representatives. The successful functioning and unwavering support of this advisory committee was vital to the successful introduction of this role.

Merging of the CNS and NP Roles

Because the advanced-practice role included competencies of both the CNS and the NP, we chose to merge the roles, as reflected in the role title. CNS/NPs have an in-depth knowledge base, provide direct patient care at an advanced level, teach nursing and non-nursing colleagues as well as parents of neonates, and participate in research and administrative activities. This merging of the two roles reflects a growing trend in other health care settings, especially in the United States. A number of papers have addressed the increasing commonality in the function and attributes among CNSs and NPs, as well as in the curricula to prepare them (Calkin, 1984; Diers, 1985; Elder & Bullough, 1990; Forbes, Rafson, Spross, & Kozlowski, 1990; Gleeson et al., 1990; Hunsberger et al., 1992; Keane & Richmond, 1993; Kitzman, 1989; Lynaugh, Gerrity, & Hagopian, 1985; Patterson & Haddad, 1992; Riegel & Murrell, 1987; Schroer, 1991). The advantages of this merging include increased flexibility, marketability, and job mobility (Forbes et al., 1990; Hanson & Martin, 1990).

Some are concerned that introducing CNS content into NP curricula diminishes the clinical focus as the need to concentrate on other foci increases (Hanson & Martin, 1990; Page & Arena, 1994). We have not experienced this in our program. The 16-month graduate-level educational program provides ample opportunity for learning the necessary advanced clinical skills as well as the teaching, consultation, and research skills required for the CNS role. At a time when the funding of health care services is very restricted and many CNS positions are in serious jeopardy, the nursing profession would be wise to consider strategies for combining forces to ensure that the advanced nursing practice model is retained and used to its fullest potential.

Graduate Education of CNS/NPs

Our discussions with neonatal nurse practitioner educators in the United States revealed that many NNPs had been prepared through in-hospital certificate programs. The advantage of this type of education is that it is short and permits NNPs to move into the role quickly to meet a serious need for medical management of neonates. However, much as this appears to be a quick solution to a serious problem, there are major concerns. First, this type of training focuses only on the advanced clinical skills and does not prepare the NNP for advanced nursing practice roles in education, administration, and research. Second, NNPs quickly tire of the stressful clinical demands of this limited role. Third, because the training is usually unique to each hospital, the certificate is seldom transferable to other settings, restricting the NNP's mobility.

Given this information, and despite substantial pressure to "produce" neonatal nurse practitioners as quickly as possible, we developed a graduate-level educational program. Preparation at the graduate level has facilitated the development of advanced clinical practice, critical thinking, problem-solving, communication, teaching, and research skills. In addition, it reduces the potential for role confusion by providing a broad educational experience in which interdisciplinary roles and issues are explored. Evaluation of the graduate program has indicated that graduating CNS/NPs scored significantly higher than first-year CNS/NP students in knowledge and problem solving and had scores equivalent to those of pediatric residents in knowledge and in problem-solving, communication, and clinical skills.

Evaluation of the CNS/NP Role

Each step of the process to introduce and evaluate the CNS/NPs was based on scientific evidence as opposed to vested interest. Surveys were conducted to determine the need for the role, to define the role, and to define the educational preparation required for the role. Cohort studies were carried out to evaluate the educational program by comparing the graduating CNS/NPs both with first-year CNS/NP students and with pediatric residents for whom the CNS/NPs would provide alternatives to patient care. A randomized controlled trial was conducted to evaluate the safety and effectiveness of CNS/NPs, the quality of care provided by the CNS/NPs, the satisfaction of consumers of CNS/NP care, and the costs related to this approach to patient care in the NICU. Surveys of the CNS/NPs and all health care providers who work with the CNS/NPs were conducted to determine their satisfaction with the new role.

Previous evaluation of this advanced-practice role in neonatology had been limited to descriptive designs using questionnaires (Barnett & Sellers, 1979; Johnson & Boros, 1979) and chart audits (Carzoli, Martinez-Cruz, Cuevas, Murphy, & Chiu, 1994; Johnson, Jung, & Boros, 1979). Parker and Cassady (1991) identified the need for a rigorous evaluation of this expanded role.

Costs of CNS/NPs

The cost of care provided by CNS/NPs was compared with that provided by pediatric residents in the randomized controlled trial. All medical and family costs while the neonate was in the NICU were measured, and no statistically significant differences in costs were found. Although CNS/NPs earned higher salaries than residents (midpoint for CNS/NPs was $53,868 and for residents was $43,439 Canadian dollars) and worked fewer hours per week (CNS/NPs worked approximately 40 hours per week, and residents worked approximately 60 hours per week), medical costs for the two groups were similar for two reasons. First, only the clinical portion of their work was costed out (for CNS/NPs, this was 70% of their full-time activities, and for residents, this was 90%); second, for the CNS/NP team infants, the 8 hours during which they were cared for by CNS/NPs were costed at the CNS/NP hourly rate, and the remaining 16 hours, during which they were cared for by the residents, were costed at the resident hourly rate.

The economic analysis in this study did not include three cost comparisons that we hope to examine in the future. The first is the training costs to prepare the CNS/NPs and the pediatric residents. The second is the savings realized as a result of the reduction in the number of pediatric residents and, consequently, pediatricians in the health care system. The main reason for considering the introduction of CNS/NPs in the early 1980s was the realization that there were too many specialty physicians being trained at the same time that there was a heavy dependency on residents for patient care. The introduction of CNS/NPs permitted the cutback of residents and ultimately a reduction in the number of pediatricians in the system while at the same time meeting patient care demands. The third is the comparison of costs of all possible alternatives to residents for patient care to determine whether the CNS/NP is the most economically efficient substitute. Therefore, rather than comparing CNS/NPs with residents, one would compare CNS/NPs with other possible substitutes for residents such as clinical assistants (licensed physicians), physician assistants, and respiratory therapists.

Provider Satisfaction With the CNS/NP Role

Eighty-five percent of the NICU staff nurses who were surveyed reported that the CNS/NP increased their level of job satisfaction. Staff nurses reported that they felt comfortable working with the CNS/NPs; that they were confident in the CNS/NPs' abilities; and that the CNS/NPs consulted and shared information with them and were readily available. They noted that CNS/NPs challenged them, communicated effectively, and gave positive feedback. They also reported that the CNS/NPs included them in patient care decision making to a greater degree than did the medical staff and treated them as equal partners.

There is no doubt that the role of the CNS/NP is a powerful influence on staff nurses in terms of education, professionalism, and clinical leadership. The positive impact of the CNS/NPs on job satisfaction, autonomy, and quality of life of staff nurses may improve retention, although this will need to be evaluated. As clinical role models, the CNS/NPs also may influence the career paths of staff nurses who wish to remain involved in direct patient care.

The medical staff reported a number of positive developments resulting from the introduction of CNS/NPs into the NICU. They indicated that the care provided by CNS/NPs was competent, efficient, reliable, and consistent. Their own role was enhanced because the presence of CNS/NPs allowed them to focus more on education, research, and more global issues in patient care. The CNS/NPs were valued by medical staff because they provided a service that the physicians perceived as equivalent to that of senior residents, who were in short supply.

The CNS/NPs were perceived by residents as facilitating their education in two ways. CNS/NPs shared their knowledge and clinical skills in patient care delivery and decreased their workload to allow more time for educational activities outside the NICU. Residents saw themselves as being in the NICU for educational purposes and not to provide service per se, so they did not view the presence of the CNS/NPs as an encroachment on their "territory." The most senior residents, who were training to become neonatologists, did not feel that their positions were threatened by the CNS/NPs because the CNS/NPs were not replacing neonatologists-in-training. The residents did note, however, that with CNS/NPs caring for half the neonates in the unit, there were decreased opportunities for practical learning experiences, such as performing procedures. Eighty percent of the residents who were surveyed, however, reported that the CNS/NPs made a positive difference to the satisfaction with their role.

Our survey did reveal an overall negative impact on the respiratory therapists (RTs) in the NICU. This group viewed the CNS/NPs as encroaching on their own area of expertise. They indicated through the survey that a physician should be in charge of the patient and that the CNS/NPs and RTs could perform certain aspects of care, mainly procedural. The respiratory therapy approach to care is based on the traditional medical model and does not include the holistic approach to care that is the hallmark of the nursing model. It is not surprising, therefore, that the CNS/NPs are perceived as negatively influencing the job satisfaction of RTs. The RT approach fragments the total care into parts, whereas the CNS/NP role was intended to provide continuity and holistic care. The RT's expertise is limited to respiratory disease and therapy, whereas the CNS/NP's expertise includes a wide variety of body system pathology and therapies, as well as knowledge of growth and development. An important implication of these findings is to ensure that the role of CNS/NPs is communicated to all health professionals with whom they work. Any misunderstanding of the CNS/NP educational preparation and role definition, as well as the overall philosophy of the approach to patient care in an area, may lead to dissatisfaction and could influence negatively the overall impact of the CNS/NP role.

SUMMARY

We have used a scientific approach to the introduction and evaluation of CNS/NPs in tertiary-level NICUs in Ontario, Canada. As a result, there now exists a new role in the NICU that is safe and effective, economically efficient, and accepted by parents of neonates and most health provider colleagues. With the financial constraints faced by health care systems, it is likely that nurse practitioners will be looked to more frequently in the future to fulfill specialty advanced-practice roles. It is an opportunity for the nursing profession to realize its full potential in the delivery of health care.

REFERENCES

Barnett, S. I., & Sellers, P. (1979). Neonatal critical care nurse practitioner: A new role in neonatology. *American Journal of Maternal Child Nursing, 4,* 279-286.

Buhler, L., Glick, N., & Sheps, S. B. (1988). Prenatal care: A comparative evaluation of nurse-midwives and family physicians. *Canadian Medical Association Journal, 139,* 397-403.

Calkin, J. (1984). A model for advanced nursing practice. *Journal of Nursing Administration, 14,* 24-30.

Carzoli, R. P., Martinez-Cruz, M., Cuevas, L. L., Murphy, S., & Chiu, T. (1994). Comparison of neonatal nurse practitioners, physician assistants, and residents in the neonatal intensive care unit. *Archives of Pediatric and Adolescent Medicine, 148,* 1271-1276.

Chambers, L. W., Sibley, J. C., Spitzer, W. O., & Tugwell, P. (1981). Quality of care assessment: How to set up and use an indicator condition. *Clinical and Investigative Medicine, 4,* 41-50.

Creighton, D. E., & Sauve, R. S. (1988). The Minnesota Infant Development Inventory in the developmental screening of high-risk infants at eight months. *Canadian Journal of Behavioral Science/Revue Canadienne des Sciences du Comportement, 20,* 424-433.

Diers, D. (1985). Preparation of practitioners, clinical specialists, and clinicians. *Journal of Professional Nursing, 1,* 41-47.

Elder, R. G., & Bullough, B. (1990). Nurse practitioners and clinical nurse specialists: Are the roles merging? *Clinical Nurse Specialist, 4,* 78-84.

Forbes, K. E., Rafson, J., Spross, J. A., & Kozlowski, D. (1990). The clinical nurse specialist and nurse practitioner: Core curriculum survey results. *Clinical Nurse Specialist, 4,* 63-66.

Gleeson, R. M., McIlvain-Simpson, G., Boos, M. L., Sweet, E., Trzcinski, K. M., Solberg, C. A., & Doughty, R. A. (1990). Advanced practice nursing: A model of collaborative care. *Maternal-Child Nursing, 15,* 9-12.

Hanson, C., & Martin, L. (1990). The nurse practitioner and clinical nurse specialist: Should the roles be merged? *Journal of the American Academy of Nurse Practitioners, 2,* 2-9.

Hunsberger, M., Mitchell, A., Blatz, S., Paes, B., Pinelli, J., Southwell, D., French, S., & Soluk, R. (1992). Definition of an advanced nursing practice role in the NICU: The clinical nurse specialist/neonatal practitioner. *Clinical Nurse Specialist, 6,* 91-96.

Johnson, P. J., & Boros, S. J. (1979). Neonatal nurse practitioners. Part 2: Implementation of a new expanded nursing role. *Perinatology-Neonatology, 3,* 25-27.

Johnson, P. J., Jung, A. L., & Boros, S. J. (1979). Neonatal nurse practitioners. Part 1: A new expanded nursing role. *Perinatology-Neonatology, 3,* 34-36.

Keane, A., & Richmond, T. (1993). Tertiary nurse practitioners. *Image, 25,* 281-284.

Kessner, D. M., Kalk, C. E., & Singer, J. (1973). Assessing health care quality: The case for tracers. *New England Journal of Medicine, 288,* 189-194.

Kitzman, H. J. (1989). The CNS and the nurse practitioner. In A. B. Hamric & J. A. Spross (Eds.), *The clinical nurse specialist in theory and practice* (pp. 379-394). Philadelphia: W. B. Saunders.

Lynaugh, J. E., Gerrity, P. L., & Hagopian, G. (1985). Patterns of practice: Master's prepared nurse practitioners. *Journal of Nursing Education, 24,* 291-295.

Marrin, M., Paes, B., Mitchell, A., & Southwell, D. (1993). *Development of indicator conditions to evaluate quality of medical care in neonatal intensive care.* Unpublished manuscript.

Mitchell, A., Guyatt, G., Marrin, M., Goeree, R., Willan, A., Southwell, D., Hewson, S., Paes, B., Rosenbaum, P., Hunsberger, M., & Baumann, A. (in press). A controlled trial of nurse practitioners in neonatal intensive care. *Pediatrics.*

Mitchell, A., Guyatt, G., Paes, B., Blatz, S., Kirpalani, H., Fryers, M., Hunsberger, M., Pinelli, J., Van Dover, L., & Southwell, D. (in press). A new measure of parent satisfaction with the medical care provided in the neonatal intensive care unit. Submitted to *Journal of Clinical Epidemiology.*

Mitchell, A., Watts, J., Whyte, R., Blatz, S., Norman, G., Guyatt, G., Southwell, D., Hunsberger, M., & Paes, B. (1991). Evaluation of graduating neonatal nurse practitioners. *Pediatrics, 88,* 789-794.

Mitchell, A., Watts, J., Whyte, R., Blatz, S., Norman, G., Southwell, D., Hunsberger, M., Paes, B., & Pinelli, J. (1995). Evaluation of an educational program to prepare neonatal nurse practitioners. *Journal of Nursing Education, 34*(6), 286-289.

Paes, B., Mitchell, A., Hunsberger, M., Blatz, S., Watts, J., Dent, P., Sinclair, J., & Southwell, D. (1989). Medical staffing in Ontario neonatal intensive care units. *Canadian Medical Association Journal, 140,* 1321-1326.

Page, N. E., & Arena, D. M. (1994). Rethinking the merger of the clinical nurse specialist and the nurse practitioner roles. *Image, 26,* 315-318.

Parker, O. L., & Cassady, G. (1991, November/December). Ghosts. *Neonatal Intensive Care,* pp. 26-31.

Patterson, C., & Haddad, B. (1992). The advanced nurse practitioner: Common attributes. *Canadian Journal of Nursing Administration, 5,* 18-22.

Riegel, B., & Murrell, T. (1987). Clinical nurse specialists in collaborative practice. *Clinical Nurse Specialist, 1,* 63-69.

Schroer, K. (1991). Case management: Clinical nurse specialist and nurse practitioner, converging roles. *Clinical Nurse Specialist, 5,* 189-194.

Scott, D. T., Bauer, C. R., Kraemer, H. C., & Tyson, J. (1989). A neonatal health index for preterm infants. *Pediatric Research, 25,* 263A.

Sheps, S., & Robertson, A. (1984). Evaluation of primary care in a community clinic by means of explicit process criteria. *Canadian Medical Association Journal, 131,* 881-886.

Sibley, J. C., Spitzer, W. O., Rudnick, K. V., Bell, J. D., Bethune, R. D., Sackett, D. L., & Wright, K. (1975). Quality-of-care appraisal in primary care: A quantitative method. *Annals of Internal Medicine, 83,* 46-52.

Spitzer, W. O. (1978). Evidence that justifies the introduction of new health professionals. In P. Slayton & M. J. Trebilcock (Eds.), *The professions and public policy* (pp. 211-236). Toronto: University of Toronto Press.

CHAPTER 12

Staff-Nurse-Managed Collaborative Care: Evaluation on a Rehabilitation Unit

Nancy Wells
Gwen Holder
Susie Dengler

The use of collaborative care models has not been well described on rehabilitation units. A quasi-experimental design was used to evaluate the effect of the collaborative care model with and without the benefit of a care manager on a 28-bed rehabilitation unit. Measures of process (collaboration, physician use of paths), patient outcomes (goal attainment, length of stay, hospital charges, and satisfaction), and staff satisfaction were used to evaluate this 3-month pilot project. Use of collaborative paths alone and with care managers was found to be feasible and beneficial in this rehabilitation setting.

The changing financial picture in health care, most notably discounting and capitated payment, has resulted in a variety of modifications

AUTHORS' NOTE: This work was completed with the assistance of Sue Erickson, RN, MPH, Project Manager for Case Management, and the Robert Wood Foundation/Pew Charitable Trust grant "Strengthening Hospital Nursing" awarded to Judy Spinella, RN, MSN, MBA, Principal Investigator.

in health care delivery systems. The goals of many changes in health care delivery encompass providing quality care that is more cost-effective than current delivery models (e.g., American Nurses Association, 1988; Crummer & Carter, 1993; Zander, 1988). Case management, in which a health care professional provides and/or coordinates health care and social services (Marschke & Nolan, 1993), is one such care delivery model.

REVIEW OF LITERATURE

Case Management

Case management has traditionally been used to coordinate use of health and social services in community-residing patients with mental illness (Clark & Fox, 1993; Giuliano & Poirier, 1991; Lyon, 1993). More recently, case management has been implemented to coordinate care of patients during an acute illness episode requiring hospitalization or spanning hospital and community settings. The goal of case management is to meet the needs of the patient with services required to produce the desired outcomes (Franklin, Solovitz, Mason, Clemons, & Miller, 1987; Giuliano & Poirier, 1991). Desired outcomes are high-quality, cost-effective care. Case manager responsibilities within a nursing care delivery system typically include (a) ensuring appropriate use of resources, (b) maintaining standards of quality care, and (c) attaining desired patient outcomes within a specified length of stay (LOS; Giuliano & Poirier, 1991; Lyon, 1993; Zander, 1988). The models using case management vary widely but commonly focus on patients who are at high risk. For example, the New England Medical Center is a hospital-based case management program using RNs who deliver and coordinate care during hospitalization (Bower, 1992; Zander, 1988). In contrast, the Carondolet St. Mary's model focuses on care coordination in both hospital and community settings, using nurses with a minimum of bachelor's preparation and advanced-practice skills (Ethridge & Lamb, 1989; Lamb, 1992).

The critical path is an important tool for case management (Crummer & Carter, 1993; DiJerome, 1992; Giuliano & Poirier, 1991; Marschke & Nolan, 1993). Critical paths are standardized, interdisciplinary plans that focus care on desired patient outcomes. Key components of the critical path include medication prescriptions, diagnostic studies, treatments, activity advancements, nutrition, discharge planning, and required teaching to meet discharge goals (Crummer & Carter, 1993). This detailed plan of care allows for easy identification of patient progress and provides a mechanism for communication among and across disciplines. Typically, documentation systems are developed to complement the critical path (e.g., DiJerome, 1992; McKenzie, Torkelson, & Holt, 1989) and provide easy access to patient variances in progress on the critical path.

Research indicates that the use of case management results in reduced use of scarce resources and shorter LOS in acute and acute/community care settings (Cohen, 1991; Ethridge & Lamb, 1989; Zander, 1988). However, the intensity of nursing care and services used has been found to increase with case-managed patients following cesarean section (Cohen, 1991), a trend that may be attributed to compressing care into a shorter LOS. Hospital-to-community case management has been found to reduce hospital LOS through reducing recovery time for patients with acute illnesses and reducing initial acuity for patients with chronic illnesses (Ethridge & Lamb, 1989).

Lamb (1992) suggested several methodological problems inherent in evaluating the effects of case management. Randomization of patients to case management is rarely used, and identifying a comparable non-case-managed group of patients with comparable risk is difficult. Existing instruments measuring, for example, patient satisfaction are not sensitive to the changes that may occur with case management. Finally, few studies have examined the processes by which case management produces cost and quality outcomes (Lamb, 1992). Interdisciplinary collaboration has been identified as one process necessary for successful case management (Bower, 1992; Zander, 1988).

Case Management in Rehabilitation

Rehabilitation facilitates the movement of patients from the acute phase of illness to the tasks of living in the community with chronic illness and associated disabilities. Traditionally, rehabilitation units have functioned with interdisciplinary teams developed to meet patient goals of attaining a functional level consistent with community living. Thus far, rehabilitation units have not been regulated by prospective payment and therefore have a broader range of acceptable care, including resource use and LOS. Collard, Bergman, and Henderson (1990) reported on quality of care in a case management delivery system judged by physician experts for four diagnostic categories, two of which (head injury and spinal cord injury) are commonly cared for in subacute rehabilitation settings after initial stabilization. Forty percent of spinal-cord-injured patients had care judged as inadequate in at least one of eight categories. Head-injured patients received higher-quality care ratings, with only 10% of patients judged as receiving inadequate care in at least one category. Although the type of case management employed was not addressed, these data suggest the difficulties in determining a standard course of recovery and follow-up for patients with spinal cord injury.

Biller (1992) described a case management program implemented on a 35-bed rehabilitation unit. In Biller's case management model, three staff nurse case managers were responsible for coordinating care while providing direct care for five to seven patients without the benefit of critical paths identifying a standard course of care. In addition to lack of a detailed plan of care and protected time for case management activities, these case managers had received no special training or education to prepare them for the case manager role. No evaluation data were presented, but several conditions were identified for more successful implementation of case management. Recommendations included (a) use of expert rehabilitation nurses as case managers, (b) full-time case management positions without direct care responsibility, (c) administrative and clinical support for the case manager role, and (d) education to assist in movement into the case manager role (Biller, 1992).

COLLABORATIVE CARE MODEL IN REHABILITATION

The literature suggests that case management is a viable model of care delivery in acute care and community settings, but implementation in rehabilitation settings has not demonstrated as much success. Collaborative care, which included the use of collaborative paths and care managers, was implemented on a 28-bed rehabilitation unit located within an academic medical center. This collaborative care model was evaluated over a 3-month period by comparing two rehabilitation teams, one with care managers and one without care managers.

Rehabilitation Teams

The rehabilitation unit consisted of two physician-led interdisciplinary teams. The teams were composed of a physician, therapists (physical, occupational, speech, recreation), a social worker, nurses, and patient care assistants. Because of the focus of the team physicians, one team cared for patients with orthopedic rehabilitation needs, and the other team cared for patients with neurologic rehabilitation needs.

Collaborative Paths

The development of paths for the rehabilitation setting posed a challenge because the care is typically not medically oriented, many health care providers are involved in the treatment plan, and the patient progresses toward goals over a long period of time. A task force was formed, including all members of the rehabilitation team, to develop the collaborative paths. Initially, the group

TABLE 12.1   Diagnostic Categories With Collaborative Paths

Diagnostic Category	Target LOS
Cerebrovascular accident	6 weeks
Paraplegia	6 weeks
Quadriplegia	12 weeks
Traumatic brain injury	10 weeks
Total hip arthroplasty	10 days
Total knee arthroplasty	12 days
Generic rehabilitation	variable

required education concerning the overall concepts of collaborative care and the use of collaborative paths. The focus then turned to reviewing data related to LOS and identifying the key services provided, as well as therapeutic interventions involved in the plan of care. Patient outcomes were established at various time intervals and developed into intermediate and terminal goals. This information provided the structure and format of collaborative paths for various case types. Collaborative paths were developed that provided standard plans of care for nine case types (Table 12.1).

Education and Treatment Plan

A complementary tool, the Interdisciplinary Education and Treatment Plan, was developed by the task force. This incorporated the overall collaborative path with intermediate goals throughout the LOS and also included detailed activities and interventions of the treatment plan to achieve patient outcomes. The treatment plan maps out target levels of functional independence of the patient, specific tasks to be addressed, caregiver training, and caregiver/patient education needs throughout the LOS. Specific areas of focus include activities of daily living, mobility, bowel/bladder care, communication, cognition, skin care, community reentry, and discharge planning. This tool clearly demonstrates the collaborative effects of all team members because all disciplines document on the treatment plan when outcomes are achieved.

Care Managers

A new role, that of care manager, was introduced on the orthopedic (experimental) team to coordinate the patient's care guided by the collaborative path. Two vacant RN full time equivalencies were converted to care manager positions so that the collaborative care model did not increase the salary budget

TABLE 12.2 Care Manager Responsibilities

1. Initiation and customization of the collaborative path after communication with the rehabilitation team

2. Patient and family education regarding the role of the care manager, plan of care, LOS, and activities required in preparation for discharge

3. Leadership in weekly interdisciplinary team meetings and family conferences

4. Assessment of patient progress

5. Analysis of variances from the path and assisting team members in designing action plans

6. Coordination of discharge plans and documentation of team discharge summary

7. Aggregation of variance data for specific case types managed and participation in path revisions

line. A 10% salary increase was given to the two RN care managers for the duration of the pilot project.

Care Manager Selection

Following interviews with the nurse manager and clinical nurse specialist and feedback from physicians and therapy supervisors, two RNs were selected from the existing staff. The qualifications for the care manager position were (a) demonstrated ability as a primary nurse, (b) expert knowledge of rehabilitation nursing, (c) certified rehabilitation RN (CRRN) preferred, (d) consistent active participation in the interdisciplinary team process, and (e) above-average ratings on performance evaluation.

Care Manager Training

A 20-hour training program was developed to assist the care managers in moving into their new roles and responsibilities (Table 12.2). The first 8 hours of training were conducted with the team and focused on financial aspects of care, care manager role clarification, use of collaborative paths, documentation tools, and the new team meeting format. The remaining three classes assisted the care managers in refining their interpersonal communication and leadership skills, role negotiation with social workers, use of tools (collaborative paths, Education and Treatment Plan, and variance analysis), and development of action plans to address variances. After implementation of collaborative care, the clinical nurse specialist conducted weekly meetings with the care managers to assist with problem solving and adjusting to new roles.

The care managers delivered direct patient care (i.e., staffing) 32 hours per week and had 8 hours of protected time per week in which to perform care manager responsibilities. Providing direct nursing care gave the care managers an opportunity to assess the patients' functional abilities and to communicate with and educate patients and their families. Each care manager was responsible for scheduling and tracking the 8 hours of care manager time; much of this time was taken on the days when interdisciplinary team meetings and patient/family care conferences were scheduled.

Each care manager had a maximum caseload of seven patients and served as the primary nurse for two or three of these patients. Other RNs served as primary nurses for the remaining patients. It is important to note that in contrast to the primary nurses, care managers were accountable for coordinating all aspects of the patient's care as outlined by the collaborative path and Education and Treatment Plan, not just the nursing care.

EVALUATION OF COLLABORATIVE
CARE PILOT PROJECT

A quasi-experimental design was used to evaluate the effect of the collaborative care model with and without the benefit of a care manager on professional collaboration, patient outcomes, and staff satisfaction. During this 3-month pilot project, the experimental (orthopedic) team practiced collaborative care with care managers to assist in coordination of care. The control (neurologic) team practiced collaborative care using only the collaborative paths. Data on collaboration and staff satisfaction were obtained before and after implementation. Patient outcome indicators of goal attainment, LOS, and hospital charges were obtained during the 3-month collaborative care trial. Data on LOS and charges also were obtained for historical controls of similar diagnoses to compare these outcomes before and during implementation. Patient/family satisfaction was obtained on a small sample of patients ($n = 21$) hospitalized during the 3-month trial.

Process Variables

To begin to tease out the mechanisms of collaborative care, as recommended by Lamb (1992), process variables were selected for inclusion in this pilot project. Collaboration among health care providers was identified as a key variable for successful implementation of collaborative care. Three process variables were measured: collaboration among health care providers, physician use of collaborative paths, and number of health care provider interactions.

Collaboration Among Health Care Providers

The Collaborative Practice Scale (Weiss & Davis, 1985) was revised to measure interdisciplinary collaboration. The original instrument contained two scales: one to measure physician cooperation in the planning and delivery of care and one to measure nurse assertiveness. The wording of the 19 items was revised to reflect interdisciplinary collaboration rather than nurse-physician collaboration, and the entire instrument was completed by all health care providers on the rehabilitation unit. Consistent with the original instrument, internal consistency of the two scales was adequate in the present sample of interdisciplinary providers (alpha for cooperation, .85 to .94; alpha for assertiveness, .89 to .93).

Physician Use of Collaborative Paths

A five-item scale was developed to measure the degree to which physicians on the team used collaborative paths. A 4-point Likert response format was used. The scale was administered only once, after the 3-month trial. Internal consistency of this five-item scale was adequate (alpha = .84).

Number of Health Care Provider Interactions

Data were collected on the number of other disciplines with which the respondent interacted before and after the implementation of collaborative care. Because the rehabilitation teams had a long history of interdisciplinary team work, it was anticipated that both the experimental and the control teams would initially report a high number of interactions. If collaborative care, or the introduction of a care manager, increased collaboration among disciplines, it would be reflected in an increase in the number of health care provider interactions.

Findings

Responses to the Collaborative Practice Survey were obtained from 29 health care providers, including physicians, nurses, nursing assistants, social workers, and therapists. There were no differences found between teams on cooperation or assertiveness prior to implementing the collaborative care pilot project. At the end of the 3-month pilot, the experimental team ($M = 5.2$) scored significantly higher on the cooperation scale than the control team ($M = 4.8$; see Figure 12.1). There were no significant differences between teams for assertiveness after implementation. Team ratings of physician use of collaborative paths were significantly higher on the experimental team ($M = 5.3$) than the control team ($M = 4.0$) despite the use of collaborative paths on both teams (see Figure 12.1). There was an increase in the number of health care provider interactions from before to after implementation for the experimental team, with no changes found for the control team (see Figure 12.1). However, this difference was not statistically significant. These findings suggest that use of collaborative

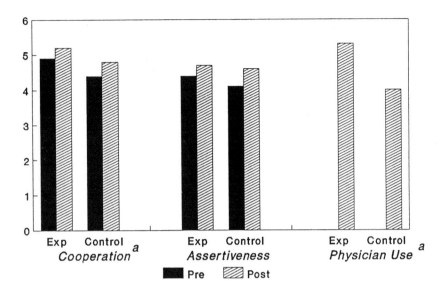

Figure 12.1. Comparison of Process Variables Between Groups
a. post-implementation $p < 0.05$

paths with a care manager enhanced cooperation among health care providers and increased team perceptions of physician use of the collaborative path when compared with collaborative paths used without a care manager.

Patient Outcomes

Patient outcomes included quality (goal attainment), cost (LOS, hospital charges for rehabilitation), and satisfaction indicators.

Goal Attainment

Goal attainment was tracked using the intermediate and terminal (discharge) goals identified on the collaborative paths. Patient variances, which provide an explanation of why patient goals were not met, were recorded during the weekly interdisciplinary team meetings. Percentage of goals met was employed as the outcome of quality care for this evaluation.

Length of Stay

Because the anticipated LOS varied considerably across patient diagnoses, the difference between target and actual LOS was used to compare the study group, prospective control group, and historical control group.

Hospital Charges

The hospital charges for the rehabilitation stay were obtained after the patient's discharge. Charges included use of resources (e.g., respiratory therapy, pharmacy, laboratory) in addition to room charges during the rehabilitation stay. Data on total hospital charges during the rehabilitation phase were divided by LOS to provide an average daily charge; this value was used in the analyses.

Patient/Family Satisfaction

Patient/family satisfaction was measured using four items from an investigator-developed satisfaction questionnaire already in use on the rehabilitation unit. Items were selected that had relevance to collaborative care. The items were (a) readiness for discharge, (b) involvement of patient and family in planning of care, (c) awareness of weekly goals, and (d) awareness of expected LOS.

Findings

Progress was tracked on 61 patients who were hospitalized on the Rehabilitation Unit during the 3-month pilot. Thirty of these patients were treated by the experimental team and 31 by the control team. A variety of diagnostic categories were included. A significantly greater percentage of patients treated by the experimental team (47%) met all goals by discharge than patients treated by the control team (10%). Although these findings are encouraging, the differences found may be related, in part, to more consistent documentation by the care managers rather than actual goal attainment.

Data on LOS and hospital charges were available for 24 patients from the experimental group and 20 patients from the control group. Data on LOS and charges also were obtained from patients with the same diagnoses and cared for by the same physicians hospitalized on the Rehabilitation Unit during the previous 6 months to provide historical comparison groups (preexperimental $n = 18$; precontrol $n = 13$). Six patients, equally distributed among the experimental, control, and historical groups, were deleted from the analyses because of excessively short LOS ($\geq$ 50 days difference). Preimplementation mean differences in LOS were 11 days shorter than targeted LOS for the orthopedic (experimental) comparison group and 12 days shorter for the neurologic (control) comparison group. Differences in LOS were similar during the pilot period for the experimental group ($M = 13$ days shorter) but dropped in the control group ($M = 3$ days shorter), with a high degree of variation ($SD = 22$). These differences in LOS were not statistically significant. These findings were not anticipated, as both experimental and control teams were managing care with collaborative paths during the pilot period. One possible explanation for the increased LOS in the control group during the collaborative care pilot is

TABLE 12.3   Average Daily Hospital Charges for Experimental, Control, and
             Historical Comparison Groups

Group	Charges/Day	SD	95% Confidence Intervals
Experimental	742	101	698-785
Control	739	118	682-796
Comparison-experimental	834	112	773-897
Comparison-control	907	227	762-1,052

the differing levels of patient acuity at admission to the rehabilitation unit. Unfortunately, data were not available on admission acuity, and therefore this explanation cannot be examined. Despite the wide variation in LOS differences, the average daily charge dropped for both groups during the pilot (Table 12.3), suggesting more efficient use of resources during rehabilitation. The experimental and control groups did not differ during the pilot phase, which may reflect the influence of collaborative paths in managing use of resources.

A small convenience sample of patients or family members cared for by the experimental ($n = 9$) and control ($n = 12$) teams completed the satisfaction questionnaires. Overall, patient/family satisfaction was high for both teams and not statistically significant (Figure 12.2). These findings indicate that although a greater number of experimental team patients met discharge goals, the patients and family members were satisfied with their involvement in planning care and readiness for discharge. Equal numbers of patients and family members were aware of weekly and discharge goals, and slightly more patients and family members cared for by the experimental team were aware of their targeted LOS.

Staff Satisfaction

Staff satisfaction was measured using the teamwork and professional practice scales of a 40-item Retention and Recruitment Survey developed and tested previously in this setting (Ames et al., 1991) and recently revised (Wells, 1993). Satisfaction scores were weighted by importance so that a score of 1 indicated equal satisfaction and importance, a score less than 1 indicated greater satisfaction than importance, and a score greater than 1 indicated greater importance than satisfaction. Both teamwork and professional practice scales had demonstrated adequate internal consistency (alpha = .74, .75).

Findings

Data on staff satisfaction were obtained institution-wide 1 month prior to implementation of the pilot project. Responses from the 40 Rehabilitation Unit

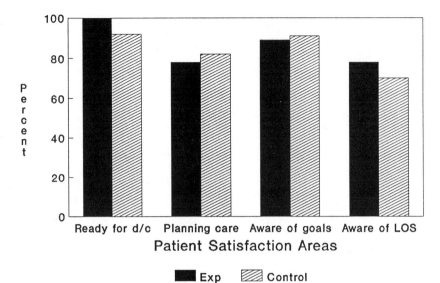

Figure 12.2. Patient/Family Satisfaction Between Groups

staff members were used as an indicator of preimplementation staff satisfaction. These data, however, provide an overall indication of staff satisfaction and do not distinguish between staff on the experimental and control teams. Postimplementation staff satisfaction was obtained from 29 staff members. All respondents were more satisfied with teamwork and professional practice after implementation when compared to the preimplementation referent. No significant differences were found between teams after implementation for satisfaction with teamwork (Figure 12.3). A significant difference was found between experimental and control team satisfaction with professional practice after the pilot phase, with the control team reporting greater satisfaction with their professional practice than the experimental team. Although entry-level differences cannot be ruled out, these findings suggest that moving into a collaborative care model with care managers leads, in the early stages of implementation, to some disequilibrium in professional identity among all team members.

DISCUSSION

This 3-month pilot of collaborative care with and without the benefit of staff nurse care managers provides support for this type of care delivery model in improving patient outcomes in rehabilitation. The findings suggest that goal

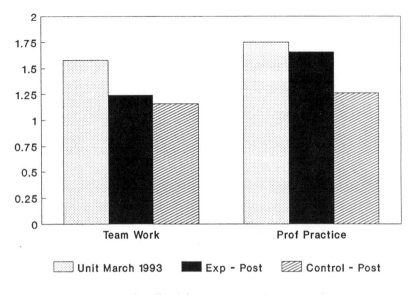

Figure 12.3. Comparison of Staff Satisfaction Between Groups
(Higher values = less satisfaction)

attainment prescribed by the collaborative paths was achieved more often when care managers were involved in coordination of care. Although findings did not support the benefit of collaborative paths in reducing LOS, it appears that the paths did reduce use of resources over the long-term hospitalization of these rehabilitation patients. Care managers did not make a difference in this charge reduction. Use of care managers did not improve patient and family satisfaction with preparation for discharge and involvement in care planning, despite the finding that more patients with care managers met all of their discharge goals and were presumably more prepared for discharge. Care managers did result in lower staff satisfaction with professional practice during the first 3 months of implementation, but this may reflect a disequilibrium in professional identity brought about by a new role with direct responsibility for care coordination.

Several limitations of this pilot project may affect interpretation of the findings. Data were collected on a single unit located in an academic medical center, which may limit their generalizability. In addition, the 3-month time frame provides only a "snapshot" of the implementation of collaborative care during early transition into a new care delivery model. Presumably, as the health care providers settled and became more comfortable with the care delivery model, provider satisfaction with professional identity would improve. Nonrandom assignment of patients to intervention groups, a methodological problem highlighted by Lamb (1992), may introduce systematic bias because of inherent differences in orthopedic (experimental) and neurological (control) patients receiving rehabilitation care. Entry-level function and acuity may have differed considerably both among patients with the same DRG and between DRGs. No adjustments were made for differing levels of function within specific DRGs, so the ability to explain LOS differences among the control group patients is limited. To adjust for difference between group DRGs, targeted LOS was used as the referent, and differences between the patient's actual LOS and target LOS were calculated. This procedure assumed that the targeted LOS values were valid and reasonable; the data revealed that the target LOS for most DRGs could be further reduced.

The underlying assumption of collaborative care is that better patient outcomes are achieved by enhancing the collaboration that occurs among health care providers. The integrated collaborative path and the Interdisciplinary Education and Treatment Plan both focused all health care providers on meeting patient goals and provided one integrated mechanism for communication. The team members reported a moderate degree of cooperation prior to the implementation of collaborative care, and use of the collaborative paths alone did not further enhance the cooperation among health care providers. With the addition of care managers, cooperation among health care providers increased, suggesting that more than just an integrated plan of care is necessary to improve one aspect of interdisciplinary collaboration. The addition of a care manager also heightened the team's perception of physician involvement in collaborative care. These findings suggest cooperation as one possible mechanism for improved patient outcomes; however, further investigation is warranted to examine directly the processes of collaborative care, with and without care managers.

This pilot study of collaborative care on a rehabilitation unit supports previous findings in acute care populations (Cohen, 1991; Zander, 1988). Case management in acute populations, however, may result in increased intensity of nursing care (Cohen, 1991) and resource use as these services are compressed into a shorter LOS. The rehabilitation setting offers a different picture, in that patient LOS is much longer and discharge more dependent upon patient ability to function in a community setting. In this pilot study, even though the LOS did not decrease significantly with the implementation of collaborative paths or care managers, the daily hospital charges incurred were reduced. It is proposed that this charge reduction occurred because of more efficient use of resources prescribed on the collaborative path.

The findings from our study support the notion that a case management care delivery model can work in a rehabilitation setting. Many of the difficulties noted by Biller (1992) were addressed in the development of this case management model. The project was developed and led by the nurse manager and clinical nurse specialist on the unit, so that both administrative and clinical support of the role of care manager was provided. The care managers were expert rehabilitation nurses who received a substantial amount of preparatory education before entering their role. In addition, the care managers had protected time (8 hours/week) to devote to care coordination. Evaluation of the care manager role was positive at the end of the 3-month trial; care managers felt the role was both challenging and rewarding.

Although many continue to view the collaborative path as "cookbook medicine," the plan can be customized to meet individual patient and family needs. These tools define the practice and care provided for various case types in the rehabilitation setting. The overall quality of care is enhanced in that functional outcomes are much more likely to occur with a coordinated plan and all team members focusing on the same goals. Data from this pilot study suggest that patient and family members were aware of the goals and patient outcomes from admission through the entire rehabilitation stay. A variance exception of the plan demands change and the development of a new action plan when goals are not achieved. This encourages creativity in the rehabilitation team to use available resources and expertise to achieve patient outcomes.

In summary, a collaborative care model can be successfully implemented in rehabilitation. Use of collaborative paths resulted, in our study, in lower average daily charges. The addition of a care manager improved discharge goal attainment. Further revision of the collaborative paths in this setting is warranted and may result in a substantial reduction in LOS.

REFERENCES

American Nurses Association. (1988). *Nursing case management.* Kansas City, MO: Author.

Ames, A., Adkins, S., Rutledge, D., Hughart, K., Greene, S., Foss, J., Gentry, J., & Trent, M. (1991). Assessing work retention issues. *Journal of Nursing Administration, 22,* 37-41.

Biller, A. M. (1992). Implementing nursing case management. *Rehabilitation Nursing, 17,* 144-146.

Bower, K. A. (1992). *Case management by nurses.* Kansas City, MO: American Nurses Publishing.

Clark, R. E., & Fox, T. S. (1993). A framework for evaluating the economic impact of case management. *Hospital and Community Psychiatry, 44,* 469-473.

Cohen, E. (1991). Nurse case management: Does it pay? *Journal of Nursing Administration, 20,* 20-25.

Collard, A. F., Bergman, A., & Henderson, M. (1990). Two approaches to measuring quality in medical case management programs. *Quality Review Bulletin, 16*(1), 3-8.

Crummer, M. B., & Carter, V. (1993). Critical pathways: The pivotal tool. *Journal of Cardiovascular Nursing, 7*(4), 30-37.

DiJerome, L. (1992). The nursing case management computerized system: Meeting the challenge of health care delivery through technology. *Computers in Nursing, 10,* 250-258.

Ethridge, P., & Lamb, G. (1989). Professional nursing case management improves quality, access, and costs. *Nursing Management, 20*(3), 30-35.

Franklin, J. L., Solovitz, B., Mason, M., Clemons, J. R., & Miller, G. E. (1987). An evaluation of case management. *American Journal of Public Health, 77,* 674-678.

Giuliano, K., & Poirier, C. (1991). Nursing case management: Critical pathways to desirable outcomes. *Nursing Management, 22*(3), 52-55.

Lamb, G. (1992). Conceptual and methodological issues in nurse case management research. *Advances in Nursing Science, 15,* 16-24.

Lyon, J. C. (1993). Models of nursing care delivery and case management: Clarification of terms. *Nursing Economic$, 11,* 163-169.

Marschke, P., & Nolan, M. T. (1993). Research related to case management. *Nursing Administration Quarterly, 17*(3), 16-21.

McKenzie, C., Torkelson, N., & Holt, M. (1989). Care and cost: Nursing case management improves both. *Nursing Management, 20*(10), 30-34.

Weiss, S., & Davis, H. (1985). Validity and reliability of the Collaborative Practice Survey. *Nursing Research, 34,* 299-305.

Wells, N. (1993). [Retention and recruitment survey]. Unpublished raw data.

Zander, K. S. (1988). Nursing case management: Strategic management of cost and quality outcomes. *Journal of Nursing Administration, 18*(5), 23-30.

CHAPTER 13

A Comparison of Program Evaluation Methods for Long-Term Care of Institutionalized and Noninstitutionalized Elderly

Juliann G. Sebastian
M. Sharron Hagan
Paula Bayer
Linda McNamara
Phyllis A. Combs

Nursing programs represent managerial innovations that make nursing services for specific target populations more visible and enhance nursing accountability for aggregate-level client outcomes. Such accountability is operationalized through program evaluation. This chapter describes the issues surrounding nursing program evaluation and presents two illustrative cases of unit-based nursing programs serving similar client populations. The two units, a Nursing Home Care Unit (NHCU) and a Hospital Based Home Care (HBHC) Unit, provide care to frail elderly clients with the goal of improving clients' abilities to care for themselves. The NHCU, however, emphasizes rehabilitation so that clients may return to their home environments, whereas

AUTHORS' NOTE: The work reported in this chapter was conducted at the Veterans Affairs Medical Center in Lexington, Kentucky, under the auspices of the VA Nursing Service. We thank the outstanding clinical nurses whose professional care and services created the data on which this chapter is based.

the HBHC unit emphasizes maximizing client functional status and enhancing the abilities of caregivers so that clients will be able to remain in their home environments. These different foci with client groups having varying needs resulted in differing approaches to nursing program evaluation. The NHCU design is based on measurement of individual clients' functional status upon admission and at discharge. Program outcomes reflect the average differences in functional status by the time of discharge. The HBHC design is similar in its focus on client status on admission and at discharge but includes a broader range of clinical indicators and uses a more qualitative approach to data collection. HBHC program outcome data originate in staff nurses' clinical judgments about client improvements in prespecified target areas. Program outcomes reflect overall nursing effectiveness with helping clients and caregivers manage health care in the home and maintaining both client and family functioning. Clinical implications of program evaluation as a method of documenting clinical outcomes of nursing programs are discussed.

Nurses commonly evaluate outcomes of clinical nursing care at the individual client level of analysis. Although this approach is important and suggests changes in intervention that may be necessary to improve outcomes for individual clients, it does not address system changes necessary to improve outcomes for groups of clients sharing particular characteristics. For example, an individual client may have excellent clinical outcomes following either a hospitalization or discharge from home care services. However, if 20% of the clients of that same service do not achieve the desired clinical outcomes, then changes may be needed in the system of care delivery to ensure better outcomes for the aggregate. Program evaluation is one way of addressing system effects on relatively homogeneous client populations. Outcomes of program evaluation have the potential to lead to policy changes that can benefit clients in an efficient way. Although nurses will always need to individualize client care plans, policies that routinize certain aspects of care increase efficiency of nursing time because they reduce the need to make individual decisions about every aspect of care for each client. Furthermore, program evaluation has the potential to suggest areas in which future nursing programs are needed.

Nursing programs exemplify managerial practices that make nursing services or products both more visible and more understandable to multiple stakeholders, including clients and their families or other caregivers, administrators, other staff, physicians, and third-party payers. Clinical programs represent managerial innovations that have the potential to increase professional accountability for clinical nursing care. Jezek (1992) explained that innovations occur when one is dealing with nonroutine problems or "developing unique and creative alternative solutions" (p. 638) to known problems. Daft (1978) classified workplace innovations into two categories: technical innovations and administrative (or managerial) innovations. Clinical nursing research has increased the number of technical innovations in the provision of patient care over the last 20 to 30 years. For example, Kelly and McClelland (1989, 1994) described the use of enhanced patient participation as a key clinical nursing intervention for helping clients make the transition from the institutional to the home environment. Administrative innovations have been introduced into nursing practice somewhat more slowly. Shared governance (Porter-O'Grady & Finnigan, 1984) exemplifies an administrative innovation with the potential to improve clinical patient care indirectly.

Another type of administrative innovation with a more direct impact on clinical care is the development of specific nursing programs that are designed and implemented for certain population groups. Nursing programs are developed on the basis of an assessment of the needs of a target population and are designed to meet measurable objectives that are consistent with values-driven goal statements (Stanhope & Lee, 1992). Nursing programs differ from standardized interventions such as those that might be found in standardized nursing care plans or critical paths (Zander, 1994) because they are more narrow in scope than standardized plans for individual clients and because they focus on a broader range of clients than standardized nursing care plans or critical paths. For example, the Respite Program in place at the Veterans Affairs Medical Center (VAMC), where the two case examples reported in this chapter are located, specifically focuses on offering one major service: respite care. The clients of this program include both frail veterans and their caregivers. Within the program, each client receives individualized services as necessary; thus nurses may care for clients using standardized care plans, but they do so within the framework of the program itself. The Respite Program is a recognizable nursing product with specific goals, objectives, and activities provided for a target population that includes both clients and caregivers.

Program evaluation enables nurses to determine whether the program is meeting the stated objectives and to what extent the objectives are being met. Furthermore, program evaluation is closely linked with continuous quality improvement efforts because the results of the evaluation are used for improvement of program activities. The most important type of objective in nursing programs is the category of client objectives because improvement in client outcomes is the reason for the existence of nursing programs. The purposes of this chapter are to discuss issues related to nursing program evaluations, to describe factors that influence the design of program evaluations, and to illustrate these points with two case descriptions of program evaluations currently in place in one agency.

ISSUES IN NURSING PROGRAM EVALUATION

Differences Between Nursing Programs and Standardized Care Plans for Individual Clients

Although nurses have developed and implemented a wide variety of clinical programs over the years (see Brooten et al., 1986, for one well-known example), it is not common for staff nurses in hospitals to develop unit-based programs. Generally, staff nurses implement technological (i.e., clinical) innovations at the level of individual clients and within the context of individual orders and plans developed either independently or in collaboration with an interdisciplinary team. The distinguishing feature of this approach is that it focuses on individual needs, rather than routinizing services for groups of clients. For example, if clinical research demonstrates that client participation in decision making increases adherence to discharge plans, then nurses might well attempt to increase participation of individual clients in their own discharge planning. Administrative innovations such as clinical programs, on the other hand, identify common needs of a specified target population and provide certain standard services that have been demonstrated to be efficacious in clinical trials with individual clients.

In contrast with technological innovations, clinical programs cluster relatively homogeneous clients into a particular program and provide a minimum standard service package to these clients. Thus a Respite Program might include client participation in decision making as one critical strategy for achieving certain program goals, but the program goals and objectives would focus on the needs of frail clients and their caregivers in maintaining clients in the home. This represents an administrative approach to ensuring that "best practices" are routinized for members of the target population and made explicit for a wide range of consumers, including clients, caregivers, other health professionals, administrators, and payers. Clinical programs do not replace individualized care but instead supplement idiosyncratic aspects of clinical services with standard components known to have widely beneficial effects. These differ from critical paths and multidisciplinary care plans (Zander, 1994) because a broader group of clientele are targeted than the case types that form the basis for critical paths and multidisciplinary care plans. To continue with the Respite Program example, clients in such a program might include both elderly patients representing a wide variety of DRG case types and their caregivers.

Program Evaluation Design Issues

A critical component of program planning is the design of program evaluation (Stanhope & Lee, 1992). The elements of care that are built into a program are designed to achieve program goals and objectives. They are based ideally on the results of clinical nursing research and at a minimum on professional standards of best practice. Despite care in the design of the program itself, it is rarely clear at the outset whether the program in its entirety will fully achieve the objectives, whether it will do so efficiently, and whether the process of achieving the objectives will be satisfactory to the many stakeholders involved. Various approaches to program evaluation are used to help answer some of these questions. For example, Scriven (1967) first described the distinction between formative and summative program evaluation. Both formative and summative aspects of program evaluation are commonly included in evaluation designs today and may provide answers to the questions posed above. Results of formative evaluation help answer questions about the process of care delivery and provide input for continuous quality improvement efforts during program implementation. Summative evaluation provides information about program outcomes, program efficiency, and client satisfaction, thereby retrospectively indicating areas for improvement.

Donabedian (1980) argued that the elements making up a comprehensive evaluation are based on program structure, process, and outcome. Others (e.g., Centers for Disease Control, 1992; Green, 1980) differentiate impact evaluation from outcome evaluation and argue that such differences should be accounted for in evaluation designs. Impact evaluation measures changes in client knowledge, attitudes, or behaviors (Centers for Disease Control, 1992), whereas outcome evaluation measures change in client health status, using indices such as morbidity, mortality, and disability rates. Outcome evaluation data typically require a longer time frame to collect; thus impact evaluation, which uses data that are more easily obtainable, is more commonly included in evaluation designs. Finally, Shadish, Cook, and Leviton (1991) noted that plans should be developed for an evaluation of the evaluation itself, or, in their terms, the "metaevaluation."

In addition to accounting for the timing of the evaluation (formative or summative or both) and for inclusion of the relevant elements (structure, process, impact, outcome), evaluation planners must decide how to collect data that will validly and reliably indicate the effect of the program on the participants. All of the usual issues that are of concern to researchers—issues associated with sampling, designing valid and reliable data collection instruments and procedures, and timing data collection to control for potential sources of bias—are also of concern to program evaluators (see Fink, 1993; Mohr, 1992). Furthermore, evaluators face ethical and practical problems associated with assigning participants to treatment and control groups when the treatment is thought to be optimal or when the number of potential participants is too small to make it realistic to assign some to a control group. Because most programs are implemented within a single institution, evaluators cannot totally control for threats to external validity. Finally, the processes of choosing or designing data collection instruments and procedures and of actually collecting and analyzing the data are costly to both agency staff and program participants. Program evaluation is therefore too costly to be undertaken lightly, and trade-offs must usually be made in choosing evaluation designs that yield information useful enough to outweigh the costs incurred in obtaining it (Shadish et al., 1991).

FACTORS THAT INFLUENCE
THE DESIGN OF PROGRAM EVALUATIONS

The breadth and scope of evaluative elements and design issues can some-times seem overwhelming to program planners. Stakeholder values and prag-matic issues are critical factors that shape the eventual evaluation designs that planners select (Shadish et al., 1991). For example, nursing values determine the standards against which clinical programs are evaluated (Lang, 1975, as cited in Tilbury, 1992). Pragmatic issues such as the cost of evaluation also influence the choice of evaluation design. Evaluation information is expensive, involving heavy time commitments by personnel and program participants alike, as well as the potential discomfort associated with systems change, data collection efforts, and anticipation of the evaluation results. Consequently the time staff spend in program evaluation is time that cannot be spent in other activities, such as providing patient care. Furthermore, implementing a pro-gram evaluation imposes change on the system, with all the problems associ-ated with overcoming resistance to change and institutionalizing the change (Lewin, 1951). Managing the change process is therefore costly in and of itself. Patients also may incur costs in terms of time and energy expended in provid-ing evaluation data. Finally, the results of program evaluation may not be positive and may in fact lead to program changes, downsizing, or elimination. Ideally, the benefits to be derived from evaluation efforts should be greater than the costs of data collection and analysis.

Wholey (1979, as cited in Shadish et al., 1991) suggested that evaluators determine the "expected value of information" (p. 42) before choosing the types of information to collect in a program evaluation. He further suggested (Wholey, 1979, as cited in Shadish et al., 1991) that evaluators plan to obtain data incrementally as the need for certain types of information becomes clear and the value of having the information exceeds the costs incurred in gathering it. Rossi and Freeman (1985) extended this line of thinking by recommending that evaluators design evaluation plans using the "good enough rule" (as cited in Shadish et al., 1991, p. 190). According to the "good enough rule," the evaluation design should be good enough to answer practical and useful questions about the program realistically. An evaluation design that is good enough to provide practical answers for program managers may not be good enough to rule out all possible threats to validity, and, knowing that, program managers must take the limitations into account when interpreting the evaluation results. The nurses who designed the evaluations for the two programs described below dealt explicitly with these issues, selecting evaluation designs that were realistic and still provided initial answers to their questions about impacts on program objectives.

CASE DESCRIPTIONS OF PROGRAM EVALUATIONS

The two unit-based programs described in this chapter are part of an overall, institution-wide Center of Excellence in Gerontological Nursing initiated by the Nursing Service Department in a Veterans Affairs (VA) hospital in August 1992. The Nursing Administrative Team, composed of the five executive level nurses in Nursing Services, developed a strategic plan for establishing a Center of Excellence during a graduate course in nursing administration (Sheldon, Burgett, Southworth, Hagan, & Peters, 1992). This strategic focus was based on the fact that the veteran population is aging, reflecting a shift in the demography of the United States to a much older population. Predictions are that 13% will be over the age of 65 by the year 2000, and 22% are expected to be over 65 by the year 2030 (U.S. Dept. of Health and Human Services, 1991). Furthermore, the national health objectives (U.S. Dept. of Health and Human Services, 1991) emphasize reduction of disability and increasing functional capabilities of the elderly. The group thought that a Center of Excellence in Gerontological Nursing would empower nurses who normally care for an elderly population to develop innovative programming that would improve the health and well-being of elderly veterans. The centerpiece of this plan was the provision for each nursing unit to develop specialized gerontologic nursing programs built on the unique patient needs and nursing competencies in each of the units. By articulating the nursing care provided on each unit, the programs would make those services more visible to patients and family members, to the nursing staff themselves, and to other members of the health care team. Thus every nursing unit in this facility developed at least one program that represented the unique focus and special competencies in providing nursing care to elderly veterans for that unit.

Advantages of unit-based clinical programming include more explicit emphasis on the values that drive nursing care and greater emphasis on clinical scholarship designed to improve patient care services. For instance, staff nurses on these two units participated actively in development of the nursing programs. This participatory approach provided the opportunity for discussion of the essential values that supported nursing care in those units. Staff nurses participate in educational programs about gerontologic nursing to maintain their clinical knowledge base and focus on providing state-of-the-art care to these clients, thus emphasizing clinical scholarship.

The similarities and differences across the two units help explain the differences in program evaluation designs. The units have a number of important similarities. For example, both units work with frail elderly clients and their caregivers in providing skilled nursing care. Skilled nursing care is defined by nursing service at the VA and is not bound by the usual payer-driven definitions that emphasize technical services and short-term interventions. Thus neither unit is required to adhere to Medicare definitions of skilled care. Nurses on both units value client independence and client quality of life. Programs on both units therefore emphasize increasing functional status of elderly clients by teaching clients and caregivers the necessary skills to achieve functional independence. Both units utilize an interdisciplinary team model for providing care, and both emphasize active client and family involvement in care.

The two programs differ in terms of whether clients are institutionalized or noninstitutionalized. One program is located in a Nursing Home Care Unit (NHCU) in which patients are accepted on the basis of their potential for functional rehabilitation as determined by the nursing supervisor, their medical stability, and their lack of available or prepared caregivers in the home. The other program is Hospital Based Home Care (HBHC), in which patients are assisted in maximizing their functional status and caregiving abilities within the contexts of their own homes. These patients have caregivers available to them or have self-care abilities sufficient for them to live independently with the support of professional staff. Because of the difference in the site of care (institution or home), patients and caregivers have different levels of control in the caregiving situation. In the NHCU, nursing staff have more control over the caregiving environment, even though patients are actively empowered to participate in their care. Patients and caregivers in HBHC, however, have significantly more control over the caregiving environment because they are living in their own homes. These differences in control influence the program objectives, the types of therapeutic interventions that the nurses employ, and the ways that program impacts are evaluated.

Both units developed programs based on hospital-wide Standards of Care and unit-specific Standards of Nursing Practice, with program implementation beginning on October 1, 1993. Both programs include specific nursing interventions targeted to meet the major program objectives, as well as health education components for patients and family members and the staff education components necessary to maintain staff competency to deliver cutting-edge, gerontologic nursing care. Finally, each program design also spells out the roles and responsibilities of staff, patients, and caregivers in meeting program objectives. This combination of program components reflects the emphasis on patient/family involvement and on clinical nursing scholarship.

A key component of program development is the development of plans for program evaluation to determine both the overall effectiveness of the program and the efficiency of the program. The design of the program evaluations on both units is a one-group, pre-post effectiveness-based impact model (Kettner, Moroney, & Martin, 1990) using the entire population of clients. Kettner et al. (1990) explained that effectiveness-based designs focus on evaluating the extent to which programs achieve the stated client objectives. In these evaluations, the data reflected the overall impact the programs had on client knowledge and behaviors. Data reported in this chapter represent aggregate changes in client status 8 months after program initiation. In both cases, changes in client status refer to the difference between the client's health status upon admission to the programs and again at discharge from the programs.

Nursing staff used both qualitative and quantitative data in evaluating these programs. The program evaluation design used in both cases is an elementary quasi-experimental before-and-after design (Mohr, 1992) because both compare changes in client status upon admission to the programs and at discharge, and neither uses control groups for comparison purposes. Because the programs were developed to provide optimal nursing care, providing those services only to some clients to maintain a control group would have been unethical. Although the two programs have some similarities in both overall program design and the design of the evaluations, important differences exist that reflect the needs of the client populations and the therapeutic interventions the nursing staff chose to meet those needs. The next section describes these differences.

Nursing Home Care Unit

The mission of the Nursing Home Care Unit, as indicated by the VA function statement for NHCUs, is "to provide 1) compassionate care to those patients needing rehabilitation to restore them to their optimum level of functioning;

TABLE 13.1   Relationships Between Standards of Care, Standards of Nursing
             Practice, and Nursing Program Objectives, Nursing Home Care Unit

Standard of Care	Example of Related Standard of Nursing Practice	Example of Related Mobility Program Objectives
The patient can expect that nursing care will provide mobility to attain optimal activity patterns and independence in ADL.	The nurse will plan and implement rehabilitative nursing interventions that facilitate optimal activity/independence.	Patients who have mobility deficits will be assisted in maintaining/restoring maximum independence with functioning in the areas of ambulation, transfer skills, maintaining proper body alignment, and preventing further contractures.

SOURCE: Veterans Affairs Medical Center, Nursing Services Department, Lexington, KY. Copyright 1991.
Reprinted with permission.

2) care that will prevent or delay deterioration of those patients having pro-
found physical disabilities and/or behavior management deficiencies; and, 3)
supportive care to patients and families through the dying process" (U.S. Dept.
of Veterans Affairs, 1988, p. 2-1). This unit includes 100 beds with an average
occupancy rate of 95% and an average length of stay of 314 days. The unit is
staffed with 19.2 full-time-equivalent RNs and 27 full-time-equivalent LPNs
and nursing assistants. Nurses on this unit chose to develop four separate
nursing programs, each emphasizing a different functional area. The supervisor for the Nursing Home Care Unit screens patients upon admission to the
unit and determines which of the programs are most appropriate for individual
patients. The four nursing programs are (a) Bowel Retraining, (b) Bladder
Retraining, (c) Mobility, and (d) Skin Integrity.

Each program has a specific goal that guided the program design and the
design of the evaluation plan. For example, the goal of the Mobility Program
is "to ensure that all NHCU patients participate in and/or receive rehabilitation
that promotes and/or maintains independence with Activities of Daily Living
(ADLs) and mobility to prevent further illness, enhance quality of life and
facilitate return to home whenever possible, utilizing HBHC or Home Health
resources and/or to a community facility" (VAMC, 1993b, n.p.). Furthermore,
each program is linked with the Standards of Care and Standards of Nursing
Practice for the Nursing Home Care Unit. For example, in the Mobility Program, the overall Standard of Care and a related Standard of Nursing Practice
and Program Objective are listed in Table 13.1.

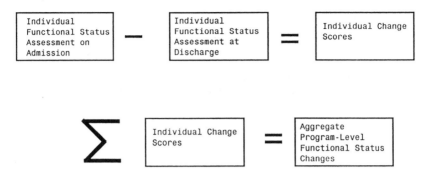

Figure 13.1. Evaluation Model, Nursing Home Care Unit

Nursing staff in the NHCU focused their program evaluation design on client outcomes and specifically on effectiveness measures of the extent to which program objectives were achieved (Fink, 1993; Mohr, 1992; Pietrzak, Ramler, Renner, Ford, & Gilbert, 1990; Shadish et al., 1991). They developed quantitative measurements of patient improvement on functional status indicators to evaluate program effectiveness. Following admission to the unit, nursing staff rate patients on a 1 to 5 scale on their level of functioning in the areas of bowel function, bladder function, mobility, and dressing and feeding. A score of 1 represents independence in that particular functional category, and a score of 5 indicates that the patient is dependent in that category. Patients are rated again on discharge using the same scale. Difference scores reflect the extent of functional improvement or decline in specific categories of functioning; these scores are summed to identify the aggregate program-level changes in functional status in each of the program areas. The overall evaluation design is depicted in Figure 13.1. Patients are not rated in the area of skin integrity, in part because almost none of the patients develop decubitus ulcers on this unit and in part because the nursing staff feel that the mobility scores account for the excellent outcomes with regard to skin integrity. The Skin Integrity Program is primarily for patients with wounds other than decubitus ulcers. Nursing staff measure changes in dressing and feeding because they are trying to determine whether programs are needed in these two areas.

In addition to the functional status scores, nurses on this unit use their quality improvement indicators as part of their overall program evaluation. Each of these indicators states that patients will have at least maintained their initial level of functioning by the time of discharge or that they will have improved their level of functioning. Finally, the nurse managers for the NHCU

TABLE 13.2   Improvement in Functional Status, Patients Admitted and Discharged,
Nursing Home Care Unit, 10/1/93 to 6/30/94

Functional Category	% of Patients Who Improved Functional Level	% of Patients Who Maintained Functional Level	Average Level of Improvement in Patients Who Improved
Bowel	14.29	85.71	1.57
Bladder	22.45	75.55	1.10
Dressing	36.73	63.27	1.28
Feeding	34.69	61.21	0.88
Mobility	44.90	55.10	1.50

write annual patient success stories that qualitatively illustrate the kinds of client outcomes that staff believe represent successful nursing interventions.

Table 13.2 presents data on the percentage of NHCU patients discharged after initiation of the program who improved in functional status during their stay and the average level of improvement. These scores indicate that a large proportion of patients improved their level of functioning and that the average extent of improvement was between 0.88 and 1.50 levels. For example, on average, NHCU patients improved by 1.57 (of 5) levels in the category of bowel continence. The greatest number of patients improved their status in the mobility category. The fact that 14.29% of patients improved in bowel continence reflects the fact that most patients exhibited bowel continence on admission and does not imply that the bowel program was less effective than the others. Six percent of program participants decreased their level of functioning by the time of discharge. The nursing staff evaluate these cases regularly and have found that these patients are usually medically unstable and no longer fit the eligibility criteria for the program. For example, when patients develop pneumonia or urinary tract infections, they may regress in terms of their level of functioning and must be transferred to one of the acute care units until the medical problem is resolved. Overall, 93.88% of the patients maintained at least their original level of functioning, consistent with the program goal of at least maintaining functional status. Thus, from a programmatic standpoint, program goals have been achieved.

Hospital-Based Home Care

The mission of the HBHC Unit is "to help veterans and their caregivers to function at the highest level possible in the home" (VAMC, 1993a). The

TABLE 13.3   Relationships Between Standards of Care, Standards of Nursing
             Practice, and Nursing Program Objectives, Hospital Based
             Home Care Unit

Example of Standard of Care	Example of Related Standard of Nursing Practice		Example of Related HBHC Program Objective
The patient can expect that nursing care will assist in meeting psychosocial needs.	The nurse will encourage patients/caregivers to ventilate frustrations about functional terminality, functional dependence/ caregiver stress, etc., as indicated on home visits.	a.	HBHC patients will be encouraged to resume previous levels of psychosocial function within the limits of their conditions.
		b.	Caregivers will be assisted to cope with demands of caregiving.

SOURCE: Veterans Affairs Medical Center, Nursing Services Department, Lexington, KY. Copyright 1991.
Reprinted with permission.

maximum caseload for this unit is 60 patients, and the average is 55, with a
mean length of stay of 8 months. Three full-time-equivalent RNs and one
highly skilled LPN provide home care for HBHC clients, with the additional
input of members of an interdisciplinary care team. These nurses developed a
single, integrated program based on the 11 Standards of Care for the hospital
and the Standards of Nursing Practice unique to their unit. The relationship
between one of the Standards of Care, a related Standard of Nursing Practice,
and two of the HBHC Program Objectives is shown in Table 13.3.

HBHC nurses evaluate achievement of program objectives by tabulating
the number of patients who improve in each of nine areas from the time of
admission to the time of discharge. The nine areas are medication compliance, functional status, number of healed ulcers, progression from tube
feedings to oral feedings, improved blood pressure control, improved continence, number of times respite care was utilized, effective use of inhalers,
and reduction in the number of emergency room visits. These nurses chose
a more qualitative approach to data collection. In this case, improvement was
not based on a difference score, as in the NHCU, but on the clinical
judgment of the staff nurses. Thus improvement is a binary measure, with
clients rated as either having improved or not having improved. Because
HBHC's mission emphasizes maintaining patients in their own homes, program objectives focus on maintaining patient health status and improving it

TABLE 13.4   Numbers of Patients Who Improved in Nine Program Categories,
             Hospital Based Home Care Unit, 10/1/93 to 6/30/94

Program Category	Numbers of Patients Who Improved
Medication compliance	6
Functional status	5
Number of healed ulcers	3
Progression from tube feedings to oral feedings	N/A
Improved blood pressure control	0
Improved continence	N/A
Number of times respite used	13
Improved use of inhalers	2
Reduced number of likely emergency room visits	1

when possible. Thus the nurses chose not to collect quantitative data about the extent of improvement.

One of the key indicators of program success is the number of times clients have used respite services. In fact, the number of times respite services are used is a proxy indicator of caregiver outcomes. Respite services are available in the VA long-term care inpatient units for patients whose caregivers need time away from caregiving responsibilities for up to 2 weeks per quarter. HBHC nurses encourage patients and caregivers to use this service as a preventive measure to reduce the potential for caregiver fatigue and problems within the home environment. Thus use of this service reflects the extent to which patients and caregivers recognize the potential for stresses in the caregiving situation and utilize the services that are available to help them. Table 13.4 indicates that 13 patients used respite services during the first 8 months of the program. The data in Table 13.4 reflect the long length of stay for HBHC clients and show that few were discharged during the first 8 months of the program. Of those who were discharged, none had tube feedings or problems with continence. This table indicates only the number of patients who improved; all other patients maintained their original status in the nine areas listed.

When interpreting these data, it is important to recall that improvement is one measure of success, although many of these patients may be more likely simply to maintain their health status. Overall, maintaining patients in their home environments while helping them enjoy a reasonable quality of life is the critical measure of success for HBHC clients.

IMPLICATIONS FOR CLINICAL PRACTICE

Changes in clinical services are likely to result from evalu; nursing staff learn which aspects of their programs are effectiv. _ and which are not. In the case of the NHCU reported in this chapter, the nurses explicitly plan to use the results of their initial evaluation efforts to help them select areas for future programming. The HBHC nurses were able to use the results of their initial evaluation efforts to articulate further the major purposes of their program and to interpret evaluation data within the context of those purposes.

Although the two units appear comparable in their overall goals, they actually emphasize very different aspects of patient health, and these differences influence both the designs of their program evaluations and their interpretation of the results. Although both are concerned with patient functional status, the emphasis in the NHCU goals is on rehabilitation and improvement in functional status. The HBHC focus is slightly different, emphasizing maintaining patients in their homes who would likely be institutionalized otherwise. Improvement in functional status (i.e., basic ADLs) sometimes occurs, but the overall gestalt of the patient and caregiver's ability to maintain a satisfactory living arrangement is the primary concern. Finally, as the nurses in these two programs evaluated their initial results, they concluded that it is critical to keep patient and family wishes foremost in terms of whether they prefer to be cared for in their homes or in a more supported setting. They also concluded that third-party payer reimbursement should be broadened to allow comprehensive coverage for patients who have achieved a maintenance functional level to allow them to remain at home if they wish.

CONCLUSIONS AND RECOMMENDATIONS

Nursing programs are managerial innovations with the potential to improve client outcomes and to make nursing service products more visible to clients, nursing staff, other interdisciplinary team members, and third-party payers. Program evaluation operationalizes program effects on client outcomes and results from decisions about the types of data that yield the greatest benefits compared with the costs of data collection and analysis. Pragmatic issues such as costs incurred by data collection and analysis efforts influence the choice of evaluation design and the elements included in the evaluation plan. Professional values shape the ultimate choice of the evaluation design. The two cases described in this chapter represent initial evaluation designs exemplifying decisions that must be made about what types of data to collect, how to collect data, and when to collect data. These two program evaluation designs are consistent with Rossi and Freeman's (1985) recommendation that such designs fit within the constraints in the situation and still provide usable answers to managerial questions.

The trade-off inherent in Rossi and Freeman's suggestion is that it is not clear whether the program itself was solely responsible for the outcomes or whether some other factor accounted for some or all of the outcomes. We conclude that the clinical judgments of the nurses help counterbalance questions about the validity of conclusions that the programs are having a positive impact on client health. Following Wholey (1979), evaluation designs may be developed incrementally as the organizational capacity to sustain evaluation efforts increases and as the need for particular types of data increases. For example, more detailed evaluation designs may become possible as nursing data sets, diagnoses, and interventions are further standardized (Bulechek & McCloskey, 1994; Warren, 1994; Werley, Ryan, Zorn, & Devine, 1994), making it more likely that computerized clinical data systems will be developed to capture the relationships between program activities and client outcomes.[1] The Bowel and Bladder Retraining and Mobility Programs in use at the NHCU, described in this chapter, may lend themselves well to computerized clinical data systems.

As the need for information about the relationships between nursing interventions and clinical outcomes increases (McCloskey & Bulechek, 1992), evaluation designs will need to focus on those clinical outcomes that are most sensitive to nursing interventions and most important in terms of yielding information that can guide program decision making.[2] In the case of the HBHC program, it may eventually be necessary to determine how often respite services are needed by caregivers with certain characteristics (e.g., elderly female spouses) and what combinations of services in the Respite Program (e.g., counseling, teaching, emotional support) yield the best outcomes. The evaluation designs reported here are likely to change as organizational capacity to generate evaluation data increases and as questions that need to be answered also change. Incremental evaluation designs do pose problems in the ultimate comparability of data across time but may be effective ways of managing the costs of evaluation. We recommend that future work examine which elements of evaluation design yield the highest payoff in terms of valid data for decision making about nursing service programs. Finally, we also recommend that nurse researchers study differences in clinical outcomes that are attributable either to programmatic initiatives or to individualized, case-based forms of clinical standardization, such as use of standardized nursing care plans or critical paths (Zander, 1994), to determine the effectiveness of clinical nursing programs.

NOTES

1. We thank two anonymous reviewers who suggested these points.
2. We thank two anonymous reviewers who suggested these points.

REFERENCES

Brooten, D., Kumar, S., Brown, L., Butts, P., Finkler, S. A., Bakewell-Sachs, S., Gibbons, A., & Delivoria-Papadopoulos, M. (1986). A randomized clinical trial of early hospital discharge and home follow-up of very-low-birth-weight babies. *New England Journal of Medicine, 315,* 934-938.

Bulechek, G. M., & McCloskey, J. C. (1994). Nursing intervention classification (NIC): Defining nursing care. In J. McCloskey & H. K. Grace (Eds.), *Current issues in nursing* (4th ed., pp. 129-135). St. Louis: C. V. Mosby.

Centers for Disease Control. (1992). *The planned approach to community health: A guide for the local PATCH coordinator.* Atlanta, GA: U.S. Dept. of Health and Human Services, Public Health Service.

Daft, R. L. (1978). The dual core model of organizational innovation. *Academy of Management Journal, 21,* 193-210.

Donabedian, A. (1980). *The definition of quality and its approaches.* Ann Arbor, MI: Health Administration Press.

Fink, A. (1993). *Evaluation fundamentals: Guiding health programs, research, and policy.* Newbury Park, CA: Sage.

Green, L. A. (1980). *Health education planning: A diagnostic approach.* Palo Alto, CA: Mayfield.

Jezek, J. (1992). Innovation, decision making, and problem solving. In P. J. Decker & E. J. Sullivan (Eds.), *Nursing administration: A micro/macro approach for effective nurse executives* (pp. 627-645). Norwalk, CT: Appleton & Lange.

Kelly, K., & McClelland, E. (1989). Discharge planning: Home care considerations. In I. M. Martinson & A. Widmer (Eds.), *Home health care nursing* (pp. 13-24). Philadelphia: W. B. Saunders.

Kelly, K. C., & McClelland, E. (1994, May). *Patient participation in decision making: Planning for post-hospital care.* Paper presented at the Ninth Annual Home Health Nursing Symposium, University of Michigan School of Nursing, Ann Arbor, MI.

Kettner, P. M., Moroney, R. M., & Martin, L. L. (1990). *Designing and managing programs: An effectiveness-based approach.* Newbury Park, CA: Sage.

Lewin, K. (1951). *Field theory in social science.* New York: Harper.

McCloskey, J. C., & Bulechek, G. M. (1992). *Iowa Intervention Project: Nursing interventions classification (NIC).* St. Louis: C. V. Mosby.

Mohr, L. B. (1992). *Impact analysis for program evaluation.* Newbury Park, CA: Sage.

Pietrzak, J., Ramler, M., Renner, T., Ford, L., & Gilbert, N. (1990). *Practical program evaluation: Examples from child abuse programs.* Newbury Park, CA: Sage.

Porter-O'Grady, T., & Finnigan, S. (1984). *Shared governance for nursing.* Rockville, MD: Aspen.

Rossi, P. H., & Freeman, H. E. (1985). *Evaluation: A systematic approach* (3rd ed.). Beverly Hills, CA: Sage.

Scriven, M. (1967). The methodology of evaluation. In R. W. Tyler, R. M. Gagne, & M. Scriven (Eds.), *Perspectives of curriculum evaluation* (pp. 39-83). Chicago: Rand McNally.

Shadish, W. R., Cook, T. D., & Leviton, L. C. (1991). *Foundations of program evaluation: Theories of practice.* Newbury Park, CA: Sage.

Sheldon, J., Burgett, A., Southworth, B., Hagan, M. S., & Peters, P. (1992). *Center of Excellence for Gerontologic Nursing.* Unpublished manuscript, University of Kentucky, Lexington, KY.

Stanhope, M., & Lee, G. (1992). Program management. In M. Stanhope & J. Lancaster (Eds.), *Community health nursing: Process and practice for promoting health* (pp. 201-214). St. Louis: C. V. Mosby.

Tilbury, M. S. (1992). From QA to QI: A retrospective review. In J. Dieneman (Ed.), *Continuous quality improvement in nursing* (pp. 3-14). Washington, DC: American Nurses Publishing.

U.S. Dept. of Health and Human Services. (1991). *Healthy people 2000: National health promotion and disease prevention objectives* (Pub. No. PHS 91-50212). Washington, DC: Government Printing Office.

U.S. Dept. of Veterans Affairs. (1988). *Veterans health service and research administration manual.* Washington, DC: Author.

Veterans Affairs Medical Center, Nursing Services Dept. (1991). *Nursing service administrative manual.* Unpublished manuscript, Veterans Affairs Medical Center, Lexington, KY.

Veterans Affairs Medical Center, Nursing Services Dept. (1993a). *Hospital-based home care gerontological program for nursing excellence.* Unpublished manuscript, Veterans Affairs Medical Center, Lexington, KY.

Veterans Affairs Medical Center, Nursing Services Dept. (1993b). *Nursing Home Care Unit mobility program plan.* Unpublished manuscript, Veterans Affairs Medical Center, Lexington, KY.

Warren, J. J. (1994). Nursing diagnosis taxonomy development: Overview and issues. In J. McCloskey & H. K. Grace (Eds.), *Current issues in nursing* (4th ed., pp. 123-128). St. Louis: C. V. Mosby.

Werley, H. H., Ryan, P., Zorn, C. R., & Devine, E. (1994). Why the nursing minimum data set (NMDS)? In J. McCloskey & H. K. Grace (Eds.), *Current issues in nursing* (4th ed., pp. 113-122). St. Louis: C. V. Mosby.

Wholey, J. S. (1979). *Evaluation: Promise and performance.* Washington, DC: Urban Institute.

Zander, K. (1994). Nurses and case management: To control or collaborate? In J. McCloskey & H. K. Grace (Eds.), *Current issues in nursing* (4th ed., pp. 254-260). St. Louis: C. V. Mosby.

CHAPTER 14

Issues in Evaluating the Financial Impact of Management and Delivery Changes

Mary A. Blegen
Richard Murphy

Nurses and other health providers are devising innovations in service delivery systems to control the costs of providing care. The impact of these innovations must be carefully analyzed. This chapter discusses several challenges in assessing the impact of innovations on costs and suggests adjusting for fiscal year changes; using costs, not charges, and using specific rather than general costs; determining effects on variable costs; adjusting for the impact of reducing charges on reimbursement; and considering start-up costs in the final analysis. The difficulty of isolating the effects of the innovation from the effects of the many other changes in the health care system is also discussed.

The need to reduce the cost of providing care is currently motivating many innovations in hospitals. Nursing service innovations have been made for this purpose, and reports indicate that reductions in costs have resulted. The credibility of these reports is questioned at times, however.

Determining the precise impact of the innovation on the cost of care is very difficult. Many of us, in the beginnings of these projects, assume that the cost part of the analysis will be the easier part. After all, we reason, we can measure money in a straightforward and direct way, in contrast to the more abstract concepts such as quality of care. Much later in the project, the naïveté of that assumption becomes painfully clear.

In this chapter, we identify and discuss several challenges to the clear determination of an innovation's financial impact. These challenges are discussed in six groups and address issues such as costs versus charges, short-term or long-term impact, total or specific costs, isolation of causes for the change, and investment costs.

CHALLENGES

The first set of challenges includes *determining the costs of care, the charges for care, and the differences between costs and charges. Costs* refers to the consumption of resources such as supplies; personnel time; buildings and equipment, including depreciation and maintenance; and the multitude of indirect costs and financial needs associated with each patient's care. Specific costs for the care of individual patients can be identified only for such discrete things as consumable supplies. Costs for services from personnel, use of equipment, depreciation, and overhead must be estimated for patient types. Although the purpose of our innovations is to decrease these costs, we can only estimate the specific reductions.

Charges refers to the dollar value attached to each patient's use of the resources such that the net collection of charges will cover the total cost of providing those services. Each institution sets its charges to meet strategic goals after a complex cost accounting process (Suver, Jessee, & Zelman, 1986).

After the estimated costs are differentiated from charges, the next challenge is *determining the extent to which modifying patient care services leads to cost savings for the institution.* To meet these challenges, we must first differentiate *fixed* and *variable* costs.

Variable costs, associated with consumable supplies and salaries/wages for direct care personnel, change as the volume of services changes. Fixed costs do not change as service volumes change, and they correspond to the ongoing costs of maintaining the facility and supervisory personnel to run the facility. Fixed costs are factored into the charges but cannot be assigned directly to individual patients. In the current health care environment, fixed costs can be 60% or more of the total cost for care. Therefore, when an innovation reduces the need for certain services, only 40% of the cost reduction can be considered "real cost savings" at the time of service. Cost-reducing innovations at the patient care level do not reduce fixed costs in the short term, although they affect this category of cost in the longer term.

Tracking and anticipating the changes in payment for the care of individual patients is another significant challenge. That is, will the innovation-induced reduction in costs and the related charges be reflected in reduced patient payment as well? If so, this decrease in payment must be taken into account when calculating the total impact on the organization's financial status. Patients have several different kinds of health financing plans. In today's environment, hospitals commonly have a small portion of business paid for on a charge or fee-for-service basis. In the early 1990s, Schroeder, Atkinson, and Armstrong (1992) reported this portion to be less than 30%. For patients in this group, an innovation that reduces length of stay directly reduces charges to the patient and thereby reduces reimbursement to the hospital. The innovation in this case will reduce some of the variable costs but will also decrease revenue. In the short term, this can be detrimental to the stability of the institution and may not be welcome. In the longer term, however, this reduction in length of stay for one group of patients opens the possibility of reorganizing bed allocation and perhaps saving fixed costs over time. To have a significant impact on the hospital's finances in the longer term, the innovation must save enough, by decreasing fixed and variable costs, to balance and, it is hoped, to exceed the reduction in revenue.

On the other hand, prospective payment plans are covering an increasing proportion of patients. For these patients, the cost savings to the hospital can be realized more directly. In the short term, the payment stays the same while the costs of providing the care decrease. In the longer term, the hospital can offer more competitive bids for caring for patients, thus gaining the contracts needed for viability.

Determining which costs the innovation influences helps to refine the analysis. Most hospitals assign costs to service categories such as supplies, laboratory, radiology, pharmacy, operating room, or a general category that covers room and nursing care. It is likely that a specific innovation will reduce only some of these costs. The cost comparisons should target the specific categories when possible. Specifying whether nursing care hours and length of stay are the only types of costs affected or whether costs for procedures, laboratory tests, supplies, or physical and respiratory therapy will also be affected helps to clarify the impact. The impact of the innovation will be further clarified by determining whether the innovation will affect costs for the entire stay or only part of it: for example, only after surgery, not during or before surgery.

Determining the financial impact of the innovation in isolation from other forces affecting charges and the costs of care from inside and outside the institution can be an almost impossible task. Within the institution, costs and charges change across fiscal years and other rate-setting events. If anticipated, compensating adjustments can be made with little difficulty. However, other events outside the institution affect the costs of care and may even dictate the care itself. Making adjustments for these external events is extremely difficult. Two examples follow.

If an innovation that reduced costs by 5% for diabetic patients was implemented simultaneously with an institution-wide increase of 6% in charges, the initial analyses of the impact of the innovation would actually show an increase in cost of 1%. To present the effects of the innovation fully, one would have to adjust for the underlying changes in the rate structure across periods.

On the other hand, consider the situation in which an innovation increased the efficiency of care so that patients could be discharged on Day 6 instead of Day 7 and in which one insurance company decided independently that it would pay for only 5 days of care. The challenge would be to separate the effects of the innovation, the insurance constraints on one group, and the potential diffusion of the company's change to other companies. Adjusting for the effects of changes in the larger environment is difficult. The occurrence of these events can be reported, but making specific adjustments would require a large multi-institution study.

Determining the cost of the innovation itself is another difficult but necessary undertaking. Questions to address include: What time and materials were invested in designing, testing, and initially implementing the innovation (start-up costs)? Were some costs of providing care increased, and how do these costs compare with the costs of whatever the innovation replaced? A complete analysis of financial impact should include the costs of the innovation in excess of the current system.

Determining start-up costs can be a particularly difficult challenge. Nursing service changes frequently involve staff and management nurses spending often uncounted hours in discussion, design, persuasion of peers, testing, modifying, and finally implementing the innovation. Nurses, like other professionals, may not feel comfortable keeping track of the time invested. A full cost analysis, however, must take these into account.

In summary, several challenges must be faced when analyzing the impact of innovations in hospitals. The first is to identify the costs for care and separate them from the charges for care. The second is to determine the portion of the costs that are variable—those that can be affected in the short term. The third is to estimate the potential reduction in revenue from decreased charges. The fourth is to specify the categories of costs that might be affected. The fifth is to identify other events that may affect the changes in costs. The sixth is to estimate the costs of designing and implementing the innovation and adjust the total savings figure for these investment costs. An example of dealing with these challenges in an actual situation follows.

CASE STUDY

From 1991 to 1994, we were members of a research team that developed, implemented, and evaluated "hospital-based managed care" in a large university teaching hospital (Blegen, Reiter, Goode, & Murphy, in press). The hospital-based managed care intervention included (a) the creation of a set of multidisciplinary guidelines for care and the identification of patient goals during the hospitalization (CareMap™) and (b) the use of a nurse case manager to facilitate the development and implementation of the guidelines, to present and explain these to the patients, and to monitor the variance of the care from the guidelines (see Goode et al., Chapter 7 of this volume). An important part of the evaluation of hospital-based managed care was the determination of cost savings from this intervention.

Hospital-based managed care was implemented in the fall of 1992 for women delivering by cesarean section. Patients delivering by cesarean section from January to September of 1992 made up the control or comparison group, and patients delivering from October of that year through June of 1993 made up the experimental group. Cost analyses had to take into account, first, the fact that the control group was in one fiscal year and the experimental group was in the next. Second, we had to determine which categories of costs to include in our analysis. Third, we had to adjust the estimates of cost reduction for the proportion of costs that were fixed, as opposed to variable, and for the reductions in reimbursement.

On the basis of the actual patient billing figures, hospital-based managed care reduced the average patient's hospital bill by only $134 (total hospital charge). The first task was to neutralize the charges across the two fiscal years. Fortunately, the administrative data system at the university hospital could automatically adjust the patient charges reported to the research team by attaching the billing codes from one fiscal year to the rate structure of the other. Therefore the data set came to us with the fiscal year adjustments already made. We were able to determine the average reduction in charges incurred by the experimental patients in comparison to the control patients in constant dollars. After we adjusted for the increase in the underlying rates across the fiscal year, the decrease in the average hospital charge was $469 ($335 more than the unadjusted decrease).

We obtained cost data from the hospital's billing system as well as charge data. Costs are calculated at this hospital as a ratio of charges for each of approximately 200 unique service areas. A cost accounting process determines these unique ratios. For our purposes, the computerized billing system provided the cost figures along with the charge figures.

The cost and charge data for all seven service categories were downloaded from the administrative database (general nursing services, special nursing services, supplies, laboratory, radiology, pharmacy, operating room). Because we hypothesized that hospital-based managed care would decrease costs in all categories except operating room, we combined the other six categories. The guidelines on the CareMap did not begin until after the cesarean section had been done. Therefore we chose to analyze only the costs incurred after surgery. The computerized billing system selected only the costs incurred on the post-operative days.

Hospital-based managed care had a significant impact on the costs of providing care for cesarean section patients after surgery. For the experimental group as a whole, charges for all hospital care following surgery (neutralized estimates) were reduced by $469 per patient, as noted above, and costs for all hospital care after surgery were reduced by $518 per patient. The next step was to begin the process of adjusting these estimates.

Because charges and costs for cesarean section change with the occurrence of complications, our analysis used the same differentiation. Cesarean patients are classified as either complicated (DRG 370) or uncomplicated (DRG 371). For uncomplicated cesarean section, we determined the reduction in *charges* to be $514 per patient or approximately $87,380 per year in FY93 dollars (170 uncomplicated C-section patients each year). For the complicated cesarean section patients, the reduction in charges was $380 or $41,800 per year (110 complicated C-section patients each year). The average total *cost* reduction per patient for uncomplicated C-sections was $521 (approximately $88,570 per year) and for complicated cases was $494 ($54,340 per year; see Table 14.1).

The second step was to determine the proportion of costs that was variable. To make these adjustments, it was necessary to use estimates for the institution as a whole. The university hospital had determined that 67% of its costs were fixed and that therefore only 33% of a change in costs could be considered real cost savings at the time of service. Therefore we calculated 33% of the total cost reduction and found that there was a real cost savings of $172 ($521 × 33%) for uncomplicated cases and $163 ($494 × 33%) for complicated cases.

Third, we calculated the reductions in reimbursement. During the time period of the study, 75% of patients had some type of prospective payment health plan such as HMO or Medicaid. The remaining 25% of patients had a fee-for-service plan that reimbursed according to actual charges. Therefore 25% of the reduction would not be charged and thus would not be reimbursed.

TABLE 14.1   Financial Impact of Hospital-Based Managed Care, Adjusted for
Variable Costs and Reimbursement Reduction (Averaged Across
Patients)

	Charges		Costs	
	DRG 370	DRG 371	DRG 370	DRG 371
Total average reduction	$380	$514	$494	$521
Proportion of cost that is variable (33%) (real cost savings)			163	172
Estimated revenue decrease (25%)	−95	−128		
Net cost savings for each patient			68	44

We subtracted the loss of revenue from the savings figure. That is, although
each uncomplicated case incurred $172 less in variable costs, the hospital received
$128 less per patient ($514 × 25%). And although complicated patients incurred
$163 less in variable costs, $95 less on average was received ($380 × 25%).

After making all the adjustments, we concluded that the net real cost savings
to the hospital at the time of service was $68 ($163 −$95) for each patient with
a complicated C-section and $44 ($172 −$128) for each patient with an uncom-
plicated C-section. Savings to the patients or the patients' insurance companies
were realized only by those on charge-based or fee-for-service plans and were as
stated above—$514 for patients in DRG 371 and $380 for patients in DRG 370.

Given the reduction in costs and charges, the hospital would have been able
to set its fee structure, for either prospective payment plans or fee-for-service
plans, somewhat lower for the following year. However, outside events inter-
fered with the direct application of this knowledge. During the same time
period, area insurance companies began reducing the length of stay covered
under their plans. Two years after the implementation of hospital-based managed care with cesarean section patients, most local insurance companies
mandated a length of stay for cesarean section that was shorter than the
CareMap specified. The results of our study showed that a modest reduction
in length of stay was possible and effective at reducing the cost while maintaining quality. However, the subsequent reduction in length of stay for cesarean
patients was due more to the insurance company mandates than to the persuasion of our evidence.

The start-up costs for developing and implementing hospital-based managed care were more difficult to estimate than the cost reductions that occurred.

TABLE 14.2 Short-Term Annual Savings and Estimated Time for Payback

Gross revenue reduction	$129,180	Gross cost reduction	$142,910
Net revenue reduction (25%)	$32,295	Variable cost reduction (33%)	$47,160
Annual savings	$14,865	(47,160 − 32,295)	
Cost of innovation	$26,316		
Payback years	1.77 yr.		

Estimates of the costs of developing the CareMap at this university hospital were done in retrospect.

The estimates included here are the first-year start-up costs and recurring costs for two additional years, averaged over the estimated number of cesarean section patients for 3 years (Comreid, 1994). The initial phase of development included 82 hours invested by the director in the development of the concept and explaining the innovation to hospital and medical administrators. Development team meetings added 60 hours. Costs for the personnel time used in initial consultation and development efforts were $4,986. Phase 2 included selection and training of case managers, chart audits, team meetings, and direct development of the CareMaps. A team of 18 people invested a total of 418.5 hours at an estimated cost of $12,666. Phase 3 was the implementation of the CareMap and included time for education of providers from all disciplines, team meetings, and development of documentation and variance analysis. This phase also included the time the Case Managers devoted to implementing the innovation with patients. An estimated 319.5 hours were used, with a cost of $8,664. Phase 4 covered the maintenance of the CareMap and reporting back to providers the success or difficulties encountered with the CareMap. During Phase 4, 115 hours were used, with a cost of $3,034.

The total cost for development, initiation, implementation, and maintenance during the first year was estimated to be $26,316. Ongoing maintenance of the program costs approximately $3,034 per year. Table 14.2 includes a summary of estimated short-term savings per year and the payback in years. Our conservative estimate of savings to the institution (after adjusting for fiscal year changes, reimbursement reduction, and fixed costs) was $14,865 per year. With an investment cost of $26,316, it would take 1.77 years to pay this back. These are the minimal cost savings.

Potential annual savings in gross costs might be as high as $107,581. These increase as longer term adjustments and changes in fixed costs play a larger role and only the ongoing maintenance costs must be subtracted (see Table 14.3).

TABLE 14.3   Long-Term Potential Annual Savings

Net revenue reduction	$32,295	Gross cost reduction	$142,910
Annual savings	$110,615	($142,910 − $32,295)	
Ongoing maintenance cost	−$3,034		
Net annual savings	$107,581		

Potential annual savings in gross costs might be as high as $107,581. These increase as longer term adjustments and changes in fixed costs play a larger role and only the ongoing maintenance costs must be subtracted (see Table 14.3). In addition, the investment costs may be overestimated because the people involved in the development of this innovation would have used at least part of the time they spent in developing and maintaining the managed-care intervention maintaining the system that existed prior to managed care. Although we realize that costs of maintaining a current system will offset the investment costs of an innovation, we did not adjust for this.

Our experience, though instructive, was not without frustration. Hospital-based managed care, the team felt, really did have an impact on the costs of caring for cesarean patients while maintaining or improving the quality of care. However, showing that clearly and unequivocally was difficult in the short term, given the necessary adjustments for variable costs and reimbursement reduction, and was even more difficult in the long term, given the changes in the outside environment.

CONCLUSION

The costs of hospital care continue to rise, and nurses, as the largest group of providers, are sensitive to the need to reduce costs and establish that nursing care is worth the cost incurred. Nurse managers implementing innovative changes in hospitals must make a strong case for the impact of their innovation on the costs of care along with the impact on quality of care. That impact may look bigger and more impressive if the unadjusted decrease in charges is used in the evaluation. However, using this approach may promise much more than can be delivered in actual real cost savings. When these impressive numbers are published or presented to decision makers, it is possible that nurses will lose credibility in the long run because of (a) the development of unrealistic expectations, (b) discounting of the claims for cost savings, and (c) disbelief of the findings overall in the absence of an in-depth analysis of costs. Using a more complete analysis is likely to result in a less impressive bottom line, but the

REFERENCES

Blegen, M. A., Reiter, R. C., Goode, C. J., & Murphy, R. R. (in press). Outcomes of hospital based managed care: A multivariate analysis of cost and quality. *Journal of Obstetrics and Gynecology.*

Comreid, L. (1994). *Cost analysis for initiation of hospital based managed care and development of the first CareMap.* Unpublished master's paper, University of Iowa, Iowa City.

Schroeder, R. E., Atkinson, A. M., & Armstrong, R. N. (1992). Pricing medical services in the managed care environment. *Topics in Health Care Finance, 19*(2), 58-64.

Suver, J. D., Jessee, W. F., & Zelman, W. N. (1986, January/February). Financial management and DRGs. *Hospital and Health Services Administration, 31,* 75-85.

CHAPTER 15

Evaluating a Redesign Program: Challenges and Opportunities

Cheryl B. Stetler
Emily Creer
Judith A. Effken

Assessing the effectiveness of a broad-based restructuring program offers both challenges and opportunities. This chapter describes one such evaluation effort in terms of (a) the theoretical, practical, political, and methodological considerations that led to the development of a utilization-focused program evaluation; (b) the resultant formative and summative evaluation plans; and (c) issues encountered that can significantly affect the outcome of an evaluation at four stages of the evaluation process: developing, selling, implementing, and reporting.

Evaluating the effectiveness of innovations in the acute care setting poses a challenge in even the most routine circumstance. When the targeted innovation is redesign of a delivery system, the complexities of evalu-

AUTHORS' NOTE: Acknowledgment is given to the jointly sponsored grant from the Robert Wood Johnson Foundation and the Pew Charitable Trusts, "Strengthening Hospital Nursing: A Program to Improve Patient Care," and to the National Program Office for their assistance throughout the grant period. In addition, numerous individuals have contributed their time, input, and expertise to making this evaluation plan a reality. Although all cannot be named, the contributions of Beverly Koerner, PhD, RN, FAAN, as the original consultant for the program should be noted. So too should the contributions of the 1990-1991 Project Effectiveness Committee members: Joy Cohen, RN, MSN, CNM, CNAA; Paul Dmytryck, MBA; Beth Greig, RN; Greg Gousse, RPh, MS; Madelaine Lawrence, PhD, RN; Jack Lylis, PhD; Cheryl Ramler, RN, MN; and Ralph Reinfrank, MD.

ation increase exponentially. When an external audience expects the project to be transferable to other sites or settings, even more complexities emerge.

In November 1990, Hartford Hospital became one of 20 recipients of a jointly funded 5-year grant from the Robert Wood Johnson Foundation and the Pew Charitable Trusts for "Strengthening Hospital Nursing (SHN): A Program to Improve Patient Care" (National Program Office, 1992). As part of this initiative, each recipient was expected to provide evidence of the outcomes and transferability of its efforts. This chapter describes the evolution of an evaluative design to assess the outcomes of Hartford Hospital's SHN Patient-Centered Redesign Program, as well as issues encountered in developing, selling, implementing, and reporting this program evaluation.

A VIABLE, EVOLVING EVALUATION PLAN

The goal of Patient-Centered Redesign (PCR) is to create an innovative, patient-centered, hospital-wide delivery system that continuously improves quality and utilizes resources cost-effectively. To achieve this vision, PCR is focused on implementing innovations targeted to redesign collaborative practice, organizational systems, and information systems (Table 15.1).

Because our goal was to determine the worth of a specific set of innovations, it was expected from the outset that evidence for the success—or lack thereof—of PCR would emerge from program evaluation as opposed to traditional research (Table 15.2). It was agreed that our evaluation design should neither create a controlled, artificial environment nor control targeted innovations to a high degree. Instead, the organization would work toward dynamic transformation while simultaneously delivering care and responding to external challenges. Evaluation thus had to occur without holding up change by prolonged testing of components.

Forging an Evaluation Framework

During the first 2 years of the grant, a framework was established for evaluating program outcomes. Five core outcomes were identified (continuous improvement in *quality, cost, caregiver/manager relationships and decision making, continuity,* and *communication*), and each was defined operationally so that achievement could be measured. For example, achieving quality could be shown by positive patient satisfaction scores, fewer unplanned readmissions and complications, and a decrease in preventable outcome variances on critical paths.

A recurrent institutional cycle evaluation design (Campbell & Stanley, 1966) was chosen that required repeated measures of goal-related progress on the five core outcomes. Accurately measuring progress was, of course, more difficult

TABLE 15.1 Grant Objectives of the Patient-Centered Redesign Program and
            Examples of Targeted Innovations Related to Each Objective

Objectives of Patient-Centered Redesign	Targeted Innovations
Redesign of collaborative practice	Health care teams Patient care coordinator (case manager) Critical paths Differentiation of nursing practice
Redesign of organizational systems	Horizontal collaborative management Customer-oriented relations Cross-functional roles Organizational culture changes
Redesign of information systems	Clinical workstation for obstetrics PC-based critical path application

than it sounded. Unlike an experimental design, in which the independent
variable is rigorously defined and the sample to be measured is clear, PCR
presented a moving and, at times, ambiguous target:

- All components of the change process could not be expected to move at the same
  pace, sometimes because of resistance and sometimes because complex, global
  organizational issues had to be resolved prior to implementation.
- Tools to measure the core concepts had to be obtained or developed.
- The hospital's current information system did not support ongoing data collection.
- The exact format for critical paths and variance analysis had yet to be developed.
- Newly created collaborative management teams were not necessarily interested in
  measuring the core concepts or establishing related goals.
- Broad parameters were set for each innovation, but participants were then ex-
  pected, over time, to help create the final operational definition or reality of each
  component.
- The nature of the sample was not always clear, as new groups and roles were to
  evolve.

TABLE 15.2 Frequently Cited Differences Between Research and Evaluation

Research	Evaluation
"Conclusion-oriented"	"Decision-oriented"[a]
"Obtaining generalizable knowledge"	"Determination of the worth of a thing"[b]
"Aimed at truth"	"Aimed at action"[c]

a. From Cronbach & Suppes (1969).
b. From Worthen & Sanders (1973, p. 19).
c. From Patton (1986, p. 14).

Our ability to define the evaluation plan further depended on the overall growth of the restructuring program itself. Not until Year 3 was PCR developed sufficiently to enable program staff to complete a comprehensive evaluation plan. By that time, many of the "unknowns" had become "knowns," clear expectations for change were in place, more appropriate samples could be identified, and information system changes had been made to facilitate data collection.

This does not mean that no evaluation was done in the first years of redesign. To the contrary, considerable effort was expended on formative evaluation of the change process (Stetler & Charns, 1995) through culture surveys and qualitative interviews. In addition, information was collected on "small wins," nursing staff satisfaction (Stamps & Piedmonte, 1986), and interdisciplinary team effectiveness (LaRochelle, Challela, & Barton, 1986).

A COMPREHENSIVE, INTEGRATED EVALUATION PLAN

By Year 4, a comprehensive evaluation design was defined. The format for the design was adapted from an evaluation proposal outline described by Worthen and Sanders (1973).

Although the conceptual framework underlying PCR was probably more implicit than explicit, an assumed set of relationships among specific structures, processes and innovations, intermediate outcomes, and end results had, by now, become clear (Figure 15.1). This framework served to organize the entire evaluation plan.

The evaluation plan reaffirmed that the purpose of our evaluation efforts was to collect information that could be used for continuous program development within Hartford Hospital and identified as its key stakeholders, or audience, decision makers at all levels of the organization. Evaluation data were to provide useful information to assist decision makers in moving toward the vision of PCR. Given these requirements, our approach to evaluation needed to be utilization focused, goal directed, and, primarily, formative (Patton, 1986, 1982; Scriven, 1967).

The National Grant Program Office, the RWJ Foundation, the Pew Charitable Trusts, and health care in general were expected to benefit from the results of this evaluation as well. Consequently a preliminary summative assessment (Scriven, 1967) was added. The summative evaluation would assess overall effectiveness of PCR in meeting its goals and identify relationships among structural/process innovations and outcomes. The summative evaluation would provide more in-depth understanding of the dynamics of PCR that

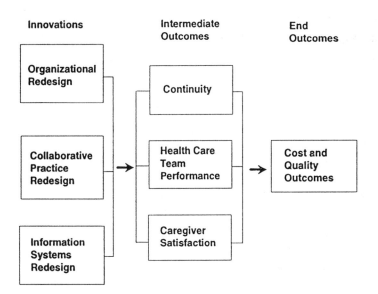

Figure 15.1. Conceptual Framework Underlying the Patient-Centered Redesign Evaluation, Showing the Assumed Relationships of Innovations to Intermediate and End Outcomes

might enhance its transferability to other institutions. However, these results would not be used as the basis for deciding to terminate or continue our targeted innovations, as is often the case with this method (Patton, 1986). In addition, given the inherent lack of control in such large-scale organizational development as PCR, summative results would not be expected to pinpoint "the cause" of either achieved or unachieved outcomes.

In sum, the purpose of the PCR evaluation was to find targets of opportunity (Patton, 1986) that could enhance continuous improvement of our specific innovations and outcome achievement within Hartford Hospital. As a longitudinal case study, the evaluation also offered an opportunity to explore the effectiveness of the overall program, as well as the effectiveness of particular innovations.

A GOAL-DIRECTED, FORMATIVE EVALUATION PLAN

The PCR evaluation plan would assess goal achievement related to

- Our *overall goal* (the PCR vision of continuously improving the quality of care while using resources cost-effectively)

TABLE 15.3   An Example of How One Broad Evaluation Question, the Relationship of Collaborative Practice Redesign to Achievement of Targeted Outcomes, Is Operationalized at One Organizational Level— the Patient Care Unit—Through Multiple Questions

Integrity of Innovations:

1. To what extent has the Collaborative Practice Model been implemented by health care teams (HCTs)?
   a. To what extent has the HCT been implemented?
      1. To what extent can staff identify HCT members?
      2. To what extent has the effective use of the HCT continued to improve?

Intermediate Outcome Achievement:

1. To what extent has there been continuous improvement of targeted process variances on critical paths?
   a. To what extent have units reduced the targeted level of variance of process components of critical paths?

Level of Cost and Quality Outcome Achievement:

1. To what extent have targeted *quality* outcomes been achieved?
   a. To what extent have HCTs continuously improved or maintained the targeted level of ER or inpatient readmissions within 30 days of discharge?
   b. To what extent have targeted outcome variances on a critical path been resolved?
2. To what extent have targeted *cost* outcomes been achieved?
   a. To what extent have HCTs/units decreased the cost per critical path?

NOTE: For illustrative purposes, only a few of the questions used at each level have been shown.

- *Program objectives* (redesign of collaborative practice, organizational systems, and information systems)
- *Targeted innovations* (e.g., health care teams and customer-oriented relationships)
- *End outcomes* (quality, cost) and *intermediate outcomes* (continuity, communication, and caregiver/manager relationships)

Evaluation Design

Evaluative questions were identified to measure achievement of program objectives and outcome relationships at three levels: patient unit, clinical service, and organization (Worthen & Sanders, 1973). Within each objective, further evaluative questions were posed for each innovation and for each related intermediate and end outcome (Table 15.3 illustrates sample questions for one level of one objective). The "Big Question"—"Do we have an innovative, patient-centered hospital-wide delivery system that continuously improves quality and utilizes resources cost-effectively?"—would be answered through consolidation or triangulation of these data.

TABLE 15.4 Overall Delivery Model Outcomes

a. Reduction in inappropriate admissions and placements (e.g., inappropriate admissions should be less than ___%)[a]

b. Reduction in variations from clinical path (e.g., diagnostics completed on day indicated in path in ___% of cases)

c. Targeted biophysical/psychosocial/functional/self-care patient outcomes (e.g., achieved in ___% of cases, for both interim and postdischarge outcomes)

d. Patient satisfaction (e.g., level of patient satisfaction on surveys should be greater or equal to ___ [score])

e. Reduction in variations from systems pathways and contracted services (e.g., ___% of all transports will commence within 15 minutes of scheduled time)

f. Cost savings per unit = _____

a. Targets set by health care team, patient care unit, or support department, as appropriate.

The evaluator's life would be considerably simpler if programs and innovations were implemented as they were designed and if there were standard, scaled outcomes. However, program implementation is "neither automatic nor certain" (Patton, 1986, p. 134), and for PCR, outcomes were often defined at the local level in terms of evolving, sometimes variable, targets. In terms of the former, an evaluator can never assume that expected changes or innovations are being implemented according to plan. This does not mean that adaptation of PCR concepts was not acceptable. To the contrary, it was recognized that unless targeted innovations were modified to meet the needs of users, their potential would probably be unrealized (McLaughlin, 1976). Still, to facilitate measurement and ensure that innovations were an adapted—not greatly altered—version of those planned (i.e., to assess the "integrity" of innovations), implementation of their key features would be carefully monitored in terms of detailed evaluative questions.

Detailed questions also reflected our operational definition for key outcomes (Table 15.3). However, an additional step was required if we were to define goal *achievement,* whether that goal was integrity of an innovation or an outcome. This can be difficult because goal achievement is often open to interpretation. This was particularly true given our desire to have outcome goals set, within categories defined by executive leadership (see Table 15.4), per the needs of a specific area or patient population. To deal with this issue, a simple scoring metric was devised. Adapted from a model used by Guild (1990), this method would demonstrate "worth"—and help the organization visualize and focus on meaningful "improvements" over time (Table 15.5 illustrates the nature of this scoring). It would also facilitate standardized comparability across patient units and services, as well as correlation between innovations and outcomes.

TABLE 15.5   Example of the Scoring Metric Applied to One Subset of Targeted
             Innovations

Indicator	Goal Score[a]
Integrity of Innovation:	
1. To what extent have quality partnerships/system improvements occurred?	
a. To what extent has the targeted number of quality partnerships been implemented?	1
b. To what extent has the perceived effect of quality partnerships continued to increase?	1
c. To what extent has the perceived impact of quality partnerships continued to become more positive?	2
d. To what extent have the targeted number of system improvements occurred?	1
Structure/process indicators sum =	5

NOTE: Only some of the questions relating to this innovation are shown. The same scoring procedure is used for other innovations, as well as for intermediate and final (end) cost and quality outcomes.
a. Questions are scored as 0 if the current score is (a) less than the target or no target is set, (b) less than the previous score, or (c) more than 1 SD below the overall mean, if the first measure; 1 if the current score (a) meets the target or (b) falls within 1 SD of the previous score or the overall mean, if the first measure; and 2 if the current score (a) exceeds the target, (b) exceeds the previous score, or (c) is more than 1 SD above the overall mean, if the first measure.

Evaluation Procedures, Tools, and Samples

Because randomized sampling is so rarely feasible in program evaluation, we tried to compensate by sampling sufficiently large numbers of appropriately targeted patients and staff to ensure broad-based and hence presumably more reliable and accurate responses. To enhance accuracy, whenever possible we used stratified sampling techniques and tools with known reliability and validity. When it became necessary to develop an instrument, efforts were made to ensure that the tool had at least face validity and was piloted to enhance accuracy. Participant confidentiality was preserved by reporting data only in aggregate form.

Initially, data collection focused largely on 13 prototype units, both because the innovations were being initiated in those areas and because of a concern for cost. Recently, the evaluation plan was extended to include nonprototype units as well. This occurred for several reasons: a desire to expedite diffusion of innovations that presumably would help address the rapidly changing health care environment, a need to obtain "baseline" data from all units, and the perceived value of related data to stakeholders for continuous improvement in their area.

As described above, our evaluation questions required three progressive categories of measures to (a) assess the integrity of innovations, (b) calculate

TABLE 15.6 Sample Items From the Organizational Culture Survey

Nothing can change	___ ___ ___ ___ ___ ___ ___	Anything can change
Tradition-base	___ ___ ___ ___ ___ ___ ___	Creative
Opinion-based	___ ___ ___ ___ ___ ___ ___	Data-based
Staff-centered	___ ___ ___ ___ ___ ___ ___	Patient-centered
Conservative	___ ___ ___ ___ ___ ___ ___	Risk-taking
Competitive	___ ___ ___ ___ ___ ___ ___	Collaborative

what we classify as intermediate outcomes, and (c) measure end cost and quality outcomes (Tables 15.3, 15.4, and 15.5). Specific tools and methods designed to obtain these data are as follows.

Measuring the Integrity of Innovations

To measure the integrity of targeted innovations, interviews and observation are being used, as well as a Patient-Centered Redesign Innovation Survey. The survey asks respondents (a) to what extent each innovation (e.g., critical paths) has affected the way they practice and (b) whether they perceive the impact of the innovation as positive or negative. Both questions are answered using a 7-point Likert scale. Because the questions had to address Hartford Hospital's specific innovations, it was necessary to design our own tool. Changes in the organization's culture, another innovation, are being measured separately by another internally developed tool (Stetler & Charns, 1995). Respondents use a semantic differential to characterize Hartford Hospital in terms of desired, PCR-related organizational characteristics (Table 15.6).

Two other tools are being used both to facilitate and to evaluate development of health care teams—an Interdisciplinary Team Functioning Questionnaire (LaRochelle et al., 1986) and a Collaborative Practice Self-Assessment Tool. The former measures a group's growth as a team, using Challela's (1979) interdisciplinary team development model. The latter, which had to be created internally, measures the degree to which Hartford Hospital's principles of collaborative practice have been operationalized (Stetler & Effken, 1995). Health care teams have found the tools a useful and relatively nonthreatening way to initiate problem-focused discussions that otherwise might not take place until a crisis ensued.

Intermediate Outcomes

Staff satisfaction is measured annually by the Stamps-Piedmonte Nursing Satisfaction tool (1986), with adaptations for nonlicensed nursing staff and non-nursing professionals. In addition, a tool has been developed to measure the level of physician satisfaction, and an internally developed customer satisfaction survey (Gousse & Schickler, 1995) is being used to evaluate services provided to patient care units by support departments—for example, Pharmacy, Engineering, and Central Sterile Supply.

End Outcomes: Cost and Quality

Patient satisfaction is being measured twice a year by an adaptation of a Picker-Commonwealth survey (Gerteis, Edgman-Levitan, Daley, & Delbanco, 1993). Other cost and quality outcomes are monitored on an ongoing basis (e.g., critical path cost and quality variances, length of stay, cost per unit, nosocomial infections, and readmissions).

From Data to Information

Because our primary objective in this formative evaluation was to provide useful information to institutional stakeholders, considerable time and energy were invested in the way the results of surveys were presented to various users. Graphic displays were used to present data visually. In addition, we tried to keep the language as simple as possible because interpreting these kinds of data was a new challenge for many users.

Because much of the information was to be used for continuous quality improvement, it was necessary to change the mind-set of some stakeholders from looking at successes to looking for areas where there was room to improve. In the case of the patient satisfaction survey, instead of highlighting the percentage of patients who were "always" or "usually" happy with their care, we displayed the percentage of patients who were "sometimes," "seldom," or "never" satisfied with particular aspects of care. Graphs provided a dramatic, visual statement of areas where patient units or services should target their improvement plans. Internal benchmarking has also been used extensively across patient units within a service, such as Medicine, and across services. We received our highest marks in data presentation for defining separately *areas of outstanding performance, areas of borderline performance,* and *areas targeted for improvement* (following a reporting format provided by the University Hospital, University of Utah, 1993, another Strengthening Hospital Nursing grantee).

SUMMATIVE EVALUATION

In response to rapid changes occurring in the health care environment, organizations are implementing change at an increasingly rapid pace. Few of these innovations have been evaluated systematically for their effects on cost and quality. Consequently administrators' decisions to implement such changes are frequently made on the basis of "limited data of poor scientific quality" (McCloskey et al., 1994, p. 35). The goal of the PCR summative evaluation is to provide relevant data that external decision makers might use to assess the desirability of implementing specific innovations or an overall redesign program in another setting. Accomplishing this will not be as easy as it may sound. Difficulties are posed by our large number of complex, interrelated innovations and the fact that it is not feasible to evaluate the effect of individual innovations separately. By collecting data on key variables at regular intervals (McCloskey et al., 1994), and through use of a causal analysis model, it may be possible to provide a more accurate picture of what worked and what did not.

Because implementation of innovations tends to be uneven, instead of comparing prototype with nonprototype units, we will correlate innovation implementation (integrity) scores per unit with intermediate and end outcomes. Given the overall size and complexity of the project, establishing clear relationships will remain a challenge. In the case that "subjective" interpretations of our data vary, the causal analysis model will provide a potential mechanism to delineate relationships more objectively.

ISSUES IN PROGRAM EVALUATION

The outcome of an evaluation can be affected positively or negatively at four stages of the process: (a) developing the evaluation plan, (b) selling the evaluation plan, (c) implementing the plan, and (d) reporting the results.[1]

Developing an Evaluation Plan

For us, the most significant issue during the development phase was the sheer size and complexity of the project. Developing a plan that could claim legitimately to evaluate the impact of such a large number of innovations across an organization of this size was mind boggling. Identifying appropriate and useful outcome measures for a total organizational transformation such as PCR and collecting the data cost-effectively presented another challenge. Guidelines for selecting appropriate variables to measure the impact of organizational innovations are available (e.g., McCloskey et al., 1994), but the burden of selecting variables appropriate for a particular innovation in a particular setting still falls on the shoulders of evaluators and stakeholders.

A second key issue was that some of our clinically based stakeholders were familiar only with the experimental research paradigm. Convincing them that an evaluation paradigm could provide useful and accurate information has remained an ongoing challenge. A related issue was getting top stakeholder buy-in for conducting a formal evaluation per se and for supporting the evaluation both financially and conceptually. Organizational evaluation is expensive in terms of time, dollars, and energy and, given its constraints, may never provide the kind of "proof" some stakeholders expect. Consequently developing and maintaining commitment to evaluation has required ongoing communication between stakeholders and project staff.

Selling an Evaluation Plan

Selling a research plan may be a one-time occurrence, but selling an evaluation plan occurs throughout the project—from the initial planning phase through implementation and reporting. When situations change, as they do in any complex project involving many people and a dynamic environment, the plan must be modified and virtually "resold." Moreover, when a project continues over an extended period of time, people tend to lose their enthusiasm. Major issues in "selling" the plan have turned out to be the complexity of the project and the need to convince stakeholders repeatedly that the considerable time required for data collection will be worth the investment. One key to selling stakeholders on the usefulness of evaluation data has been showing users how to link data about staff satisfaction, leadership, team development, and customer satisfaction to cost and quality outcomes in their particular domain (see Shortell et al., 1992).

Implementing an Evaluation Plan

Two major issues have been identified during the implementation phase. The first is learning how best to collect some kinds of data so that too-frequent surveying or interviewing of staff can be avoided. The second relates to finding the necessary resources both now (while the project staff is on board) and in the future (when data collection is integrated into the organizational structure) to organize data from multiple sources being tracked over a 4-year period. This has meant organizing a limited number of dedicated program grant staff to coordinate and do the initial work and modeling of evaluation systems, and then gradually restructuring, educating, and supporting various parts of the operating system to assume responsibility for ongoing data collection, analysis, and reporting.

Reporting the Results

Our goal has been to make certain that all constituencies receive the evaluative information that will be most helpful to them in a format they can understand. Consistent with the project's emphasis on continuous quality improvement, feedback is solicited routinely about the nature of reports that have been provided so that improvements can be made along the way. A challenge of the reporting component of PCR evaluation is the sheer volume of data being collected! We have tried to present data in short, concise, and user-friendly formats. Yet a balance must be struck between parsimony and loss of potentially insightful information.

SUMMARY

Assessing the success of an organizational transformation is a complex activity. The approach chosen to assess the success of PCR at Hartford Hospital has focused on monitoring improvement, over time, relative to the achievement of continuously evolving and targeted goals. Although this dynamic design does not have the "causal" strength of a highly controlled experimental study, it does have the "reality-based" strength of reflecting real change within the real world of organizational operations and redesign.

Both the level of goal achievement and relationships among the multifaceted components of this planned organizational change are being determined through an accumulation or preponderance of evidence (Smith, 1981). Multiple sets of quantitative and qualitative data have been collected, ranging from quantitative perceptions of affected groups and individuals, to qualitative descriptions of critical events, case studies, and "small wins," to continuous, measurable improvements in structure, process, and outcome indicators. Progress on individual components of redesign, such as implementation of health care teams or customer-oriented relationships, is being assessed and used to enhance or modify each innovation. Hypothesized relationships between structure and/or process and outcome are also being explored. However, in the end, an answer to the "Big Question" of whether Hartford Hospital has achieved its vision will come from interpreting the gestalt of evidence as well as its credibility to individuals for whom the answer is significant.

NOTE

1. These issues were identified within the context of a Delphi process involving project evaluators/directors of six hospitals participating in the Robert Wood Johnson Foundation/the Pew Charitable Trusts' Strengthening Hospital Nursing Grant Projects (National Program Office, 1992). The issues cited here reflect only Hartford Hospital's evaluation.

REFERENCES

Campbell, D. T., & Stanley, J. C. (1966). *Experimental and quasi-experimental designs for research.* Chicago: Rand McNally.

Challela, M. (1979). The interdisciplinary team: A role definition for nursing. *Image, 11*(1), 9-15.

Cronbach, L. J., & Suppes, P. (1969). *Research for tomorrow's schools: Disciplined inquiry of education.* New York: Macmillan.

Gerteis, M., Edgman-Levitan, S., Daley, J., & Delbanco, T. L. (1993). *Through the patient's eyes: Understanding and promoting patient-centered care.* San Francisco: Jossey-Bass.

Gousse, G., & Schickler, J. (1995). Quality partnerships. In C. B. Stetler & M. P. Charns (Eds.), *Collaboration in health care: Hartford Hospital's journey in changing management and practice* (pp. 149-168). Chicago: American Hospital Publishing.

Guild, P. A. (1990). Goal-oriented evaluation as a program management tool. *American Journal of Health Promotion, 4,* 296-301.

LaRochelle, D., Challela, M., & Barton, A. (1986). *An interdisciplinary team functioning questionnaire.* Unpublished manuscript.

McCloskey, J. C., Mass, M., Huber, D. G., Kasparek, A., Specht, J., Ramler, C., Watson, C., Blegen, M., Delaney, C., Ellerbe, S., Etscheidt, C., Gongaware, C., Johnson, M., Kelly, K., Mehmert, P., & Clougherty, J. (1994). Nursing management innovations: A need for systematic evaluation. *Nursing Economics, 12*(1), 35-44.

McLaughlin, M. (1976). Implementation as mutual adaptation. In W. Williams & R. F. Elmore (Eds.), *Social program implementation* (pp. 167-180). New York: Academic Press.

National Program Office. (1992). *Strengthening hospital nursing: A program to improve patient care, gaining momentum: A progress report.* St. Petersburg, FL: Author.

Patton, M. Q. (1982). *Practical evaluation.* Beverly Hills, CA: Sage.

Patton, M. Q. (1986). *Utilization-focused evaluation* (2nd ed.). Beverly Hills, CA: Sage.

Scriven, M. (1967). The methodology of evaluation. In R. W. Tyler, R. M. Gagne, & M. Scriven (Eds.), *Perspectives of curriculum evaluation* (pp. 39-83). Chicago: Rand McNally.

Shortell, S. M., Zimmerman, J. E., Gillies, R. R., Duffy, J., Devers, K. J., Rousseau, D. M., & Knaus, W. A. (1992). Continuously improving patient care: Practical lessons and an assessment tool from the National ICU Study. *Quality Review Bulletin, 18,* 150-155.

Smith, N. L. (1981). Creating alternative methods for educational evaluation. In N. L. Smith (Ed.), *Federal evaluation efforts to develop new evaluation methods* (pp. 84-97). San Francisco: Jossey-Bass.

Stamps, P. L., & Piedmonte, E. (1986). *Nurses and work satisfaction: An index for measurement.* Ann Arbor, MI: Health Administration Press.

Stetler, C., & Charns, M. (Eds.). (1995). *Collaboration in health care: Hartford Hospital's journey in changing management and practice.* Chicago: American Hospital Publishing.

Stetler, C., & Effken, J. (1995). Redesign of collaboration in practice: From a sound foundation to beginning integration. In C. B. Stetler & M. P. Charns (Eds.), *Collaboration in health care: Hartford Hospital's journey in changing management and practice* (pp. 201-215). Chicago: American Hospital Publishing.

Worthen, B. R., & Sanders, J. R. (1973). *Educational evaluation: Theory and practice.* Belmont, CA: Wadsworth.

Index

About the Editors

Kathleen C. Kelly, PhD, RN, is Assistant Professor at the College of Nursing, University of Iowa, Iowa City, where she teaches two graduate courses in the master's curriculum: Nursing Administration II: Process, Roles, and Strategies, and Case Management in Health Delivery Systems. In addition, she directs the College of Nursing's Office of Continuing Education and is Adjunct Associate Director of Nursing, St. Luke's Hospital, Cedar Rapids, Iowa. Her career has included clinical, academic, consultation, and administration roles. She served in clinical nurse specialist and ambulatory nurse management roles at the University of Iowa Hospitals and Clinics and for 8 years was Executive Director of the Visiting Nurse Association of Johnson County, Iowa. She served as a member of the Board of Directors of the National Association for Home Care and is currently a member of the Executive Committee of the ANA Council for Professional Development and Education. This volume is the fourth to be edited by her, and she has been a member of the Series on Nursing Administration Board of Directors since the development of the second volume. Her research foci are health care systems and client participation in decision making as they relate to achieving continuity of care based on need rather than resources. Recent publications address the nursing perspective on the Medical Outcomes Studies and adjunct executive appointments for faculty in health care provider organizations.

Meridean L. Maas, PhD, RN, FAAN, is Professor, College of Nursing, University of Iowa, Iowa City, and Adjunct Associate Executive in Nursing, Iowa Veterans Home, Marshalltown, Iowa. She teaches in the Nursing Service Administration graduate programs for master's and doctoral students, specializing in long-term care administration. She is active in a number of professional organizations, including the American Nurses Association and the American Academy of Nursing. Prior to her academic career, she had a long nursing practice career during which she administered a nursing department and school of nursing in an acute care hospital, held staff development and supervisory positions in hospitals, and worked as a clinical specialist and administrator in long-term care. Her research focuses on the development and testing of nursing management and clinical interventions and classifications of standardized languages for nursing diagnoses, interventions, and nursing-sensitive patient outcomes. She has been principal investigator for research that has generated more than $3 million dollars in external funding. She was principal investigator for one of the first federally funded grants awarded to a nonacademic institution to describe and evaluate the effects of implementation of a nursing shared-governance model on patients and staff, "Nurse Autonomy and Patient Welfare." Currently she is Principal Investigator for a National Institute of Nursing (NINR) funded 4-year grant to test the effects of a Family Involvement in Care nursing intervention for family members of persons with Alzheimer's disease (AD) who are institutionalized on family members, staff, and AD patients. She also is Coprincipal Investigator (Marion Johnson, Principal Investigator) for a 4-year NINR-funded study to develop and test a Nursing-Sensitive Outcomes Classification (NOC). She has numerous data-based and scholarly publications, including several books and numerous journal articles and book chapters.

About the Contributors

Ida M. Androwich, PhD, RN, Associate Professor and Administrative Director, Nursing Education & Support Services, Loyola University Medical Center, Maywood Illinois.

Paula Bayer, BSN, RN, is Nurse Manager, Nursing Home Care Unit, Veterans Affairs Medical Center, Lexington, Kentucky.

Mary A. Blegen, PhD, RN, is Associate Professor, College of Nursing, University of Iowa, and Adjunct Clinical Staff, Case Management, University of Iowa Hospitals and Clinics, Iowa City, Iowa.

Greg Clancy, RN, BSN, is Nurse Case Manager, Critical Care Division, University of Iowa Hospitals and Clinics, Iowa City, Iowa.

Jennifer Clougherty, BSBE, is Program Associate, Nursing Service Administration, College of Nursing, University of Iowa, Iowa City, Iowa.

Mary S. Collins, PhD, RN, is Dean and Associate Professor, Decker School of Nursing, Binghamton University, Binghamton, New York.

Phyllis A. Combs, MN, RN, is Program Director of Hospital Based Home Care at the Veterans Affairs Medical Center, Lexington, Kentucky.

Reni Courtney, RN, CFNP, PhD, is Project Director of the Partnership Action for Healthy Communities Project and Specialist at the University of Texas at Arlington School of Nursing, Arlington, Texas.

Emily Creer, MA, is Data Coordinator for the Patient-Centered Redesign Program at Hartford Hospital, Hartford, Connecticut.

Connie Delaney, PhD, RN, is Associate Professor, College of Nursing, University of Iowa, and Adjunct Clinical Staff, Informatics, University of Iowa Hospitals and Clinics, Iowa City, Iowa.

Susie Dengler, MSN, RN, is Clinical Nurse Specialist, Rehabilitation Unit, Vanderbilt University Medical Center, Vanderbilt, Tennessee.

Judith A. Effken, PhD, RN, CNA, is Administrative Systems Coordinator for the Patient-Centered Redesign Program at Hartford Hospital, Hartford, Connecticut.

Suellyn Ellerbe, MN, RN, is Vice President of Nursing, Mercy Hospital, Davenport, Iowa.

Carlie Etscheidt, MS, RN, is Director of Quality Improvement and Special Care Services, Mercy Medical Center, Cedar Rapids, Iowa.

Carole Gongaware, MSN, RN, is Vice President of Patient Services, Genesis Medical Center, Davenport, Iowa.

Colleen J. Goode, RN, PhD, CNAA, is Senior Associate to the Director of Nursing and Patient Care Services, University of Iowa Hospitals and Clinics, Iowa City, Iowa.

Sheila A. Haas, PhD, RN, is Professor and Department Chair, Community and Administrative Nursing, Loyola University, Chicago, Illinois.

M. Sharron Hagan, MSN, RN, is Supervisor, Nursing Home Care Unit, Veterans Affairs Medical Center, Lexington, Kentucky.

Teresa Hamilton, RN, BSN, is Nurse Case Manager, OB/GYN Division, University of Iowa Hospitals and Clinics, Iowa City, Iowa.

Almira T. Hinton, RN, BSN, is Nurse Case Manager, OB/GYN Division, University of Iowa Hospitals and Clinics, Iowa City, Iowa.

Gwen Holder, MSN, RN, is Manager, Rehabilitation Unit, Vanderbilt University Medical Center, Vanderbilt, Tennessee.

Diane Gardner Huber, PhD, RN, is Associate Professor, College of Nursing, University of Iowa, and Adjunct Associate Director, Mercy Hospital, Iowa City, Iowa.

Vicki Ibarra, RN, MA, is Case Management/Project Manager, University of Iowa Hospitals and Clinics, Iowa City, Iowa.

Marion R. Johnson, PhD, RN, is Associate Professor, College of Nursing, University of Iowa, and Adjunct Associate Director of Nursing, Mercy Medical Center, Cedar Rapids, Iowa.

Ann Kasparek, MA, RN, is Director of Patient Care Management and Medical Services, Mercy Medical Center, Cedar Rapids, Iowa.

Vicki L. Kraus, MS, RN, CS, is Clinical Nurse Specialist, Department of Nursing, University of Iowa Hospitals and Clinics, and Doctoral Candidate, College of Nursing, University of Iowa, Iowa City, Iowa.

Virginia L. Maturen, MSN, MM, RN, is Executive Director of VNA *First,* Berwyn, Illinois.

Joanne Comi McCloskey, PhD, RN, FAAN, is Distinguished Professor of Nursing, College of Nursing, University of Iowa, and Adjunct Associate Director of Nursing, University of Iowa Hospitals and Clinics, Iowa City, Iowa.

Linda McNamara, BSN, RN, is Nurse Manager, Nursing Home Care Unit, Veterans Affairs Medical Center, Lexington, Kentucky.

Peg Mehmert, MSN, RN, is Director of Nursing Practice/Systems Integration, Genesis Medical Center, Davenport, Iowa.

Roxanne Mills, RN, MA Candidate, is Nurse Case Manager, OB/GYN Division, University of Iowa Hospitals and Clinics, Iowa City, Iowa.

Alba Mitchell-DiCenso, RN, MSc, PhD, is Associate Professor, School of Nursing, McMaster University, Hamilton, Ontario, Canada, and Career Scientist, Ontario Ministry of Health, Toronto, Ontario, Canada.

Richard Murphy, MBA, is Associate Director, Financial Management and Control, University of Iowa Hospitals and Clinics, Iowa City, Iowa.

Elizabeth Parietti, EdD, RN, is a former Associate Professor, Decker School of Nursing, Binghamton University, Binghamton, New York.

Janet Pinelli, RN, MScN, DNS Candidate, is Associate Professor, School of Nursing, McMaster University, and Clinical Nurse Specialist/Neonatal Practitioner, McMaster Division, Chedoke-McMaster Hospitals, Hamilton, Ontario, Canada.

Cheryl L. Ramler, PhD, RN, is Program Assistant and Doctoral Candidate, College of Nursing, University of Iowa, Iowa City, Iowa and student in nurse anesthesia program, University of Iowa.

Jan Reighard, RN, BSN, is Nurse Case Manager, OB/GYN Division, University of Iowa Hospitals and Clinics, Iowa City, Iowa.

Juliann G. Sebastian, PhD, RN, CS, is Associate Professor and Director of Clinical Affairs, University of Kentucky College of Nursing, Lexington, Kentucky.

Doris Southwell is Project Coordinator, School of Nursing, McMaster University, Hamilton, Ontario, Canada.

Janet Pringle Specht, MA, RNC, is a Program Assistant and Doctoral Candidate in the College of Nursing, University of Iowa, Iowa City, Iowa.

Gale A. Spencer, PhD, RN, is Associate Professor and Director of the Center for Nursing Research, Decker School of Nursing, Binghamton University, Binghamton, New York.

Victoria M. Steelman, MA, PhD Candidate, RN, is Clinical Nurse Specialist, Intensive and Surgical Services Nursing, University of Iowa Hospitals and Clinics, Iowa City, Iowa.

Cheryl B. Stetler, PhD, RN, FAAN, is Project Director for the Patient-Centered Redesign Program at Hartford Hospital, Hartford, Connecticut.

Marita G. Titler, PhD, RN, FAAN, is Associate Director, Office of Outcomes Evaluation and Management, and Nursing Research, University of Iowa Hospitals and Clinics, Iowa City, Iowa.

Jean Barry Walker, RN, MS, CNA, is Clinical Director, Medical Nursing Division, University of Iowa Hospitals and Clinics, Iowa City, Iowa.

Jean A. Walters, MS, RN, was Vice President of Patient Care Services, Froedtert Memorial Lutheran Hospital, Milwaukee, Wisconsin.

Carol Watson, PhD, RN, is Vice President of Patient Care, Mercy Medical Center, Cedar Rapids, Iowa.

Nancy Wells, DNSc, RN, is Director of Nursing Research, Vanderbilt University Medical Center, Vanderbilt, Tennessee.